T0021679

CHAKRAS, FOOD, AND YOU

TAP YOUR INDIVIDUAL ENERGY SYSTEM
for HEALTH, HEALING,
and HARMONIOUS WEIGHT

Cyndi Dale and Dana Childs

ST. MARTIN'S
ESSENTIALS
NEW YORK

First published in the United States by St. Martin's Essentials, an imprint of St. Martin's Publishing Group.

www.stmartins.com

Designed by Steven Seighman

Cover photographs: tomato © StudioPhotoDFlorez/Shutterstock.com; orange © Photoongraphy/Shutterstock.com; yellow pepper © Bozena Fulawka/Shutterstock.com; broccoli © Mirra/Shutterstock.com; blueberries © Photoongraphy/Shutterstock.com; red cabbage © StudioPhotoDFlorez/Shutterstock.com; garlic © Jacek Fulawka/Shutterstock.com; black beans © onair/Shutterstock.com; turmeric © Num LPPHOTO/Shutterstock.com; almonds © art_of_galaxy/Shutterstock.com; dragon fruit © Nataly Studio/Shutterstock.com; water © CK Foto/Shutterstock.com

Library of Congress Cataloging-in-Publication Data

Names: Dale, Cyndi, author. | Childs, Dana, author.
Title: Chakras, food, and you: tap your individual energy system for health, healing, and harmonious weight / Cyndi Dale and Dana Childs.
Description: First edition. | New York: St. Martin's Essentials, 2021. | Includes bibliographical references.
Identifiers: LCCN 2021008177 | ISBN 9781250790675 (hardcover) | ISBN 9781250790682 (ebook)
Subjects: LCSH: Chakras. | Food—Miscellanea. | Health.
Classification: LCC BF1442.C53 D353 2021 | DDC 131—dc23
LC record available at https://lccn.loc.gov/2021008177

Our books may be purchased in bulk for promotional, educational, or business use. Please contact your local bookseller or the Macmillan Corporate and Premium Sales Department at 1-800-221-7945, extension 5442, or by email at MacmillanSpecialMarkets@macmillan.com.

First Edition: 2021

10 9 8 7 6 5 4 3 2 1

To all those who have fed us

CONTENTS

INTRODUCTION

Tired of trying every diet system and supplement on the shelf and still not getting results? Feeling discouraged, guilty, or overwhelmed because the foods on the most recent trendy plan don't appeal to you? Worse, are you sick of eating all the so-called healthy foods, only to gain weight while your friend chomps pizza and fries—and remains slim? Or the reverse—eating all the foods you can fit in your mouth to put weight on with no luck?

We've been there. In fact, we grew so weary of chasing health and losing the battle with weight, that we combined our collective experience and expertise to create an innovative approach to health and wellness. It's unlike anything else you've seen. It's been working for us and our clients. And it's just too good to *not* share. The secret? It's based on *chakras*.

This unique process synchronizes your *choices* with your chakras—your *single* most important chakra, to be exact—so you can reshape your body and, therefore, your entire well-being. In fact, we believe that by customizing your food and supplementation choices to your most vital chakra you can achieve optimum health. In this way, you encourage healing from issues impacting your wellness. If you need a weight change, you'll notice the difference—not because you're "dieting," but because you're feeding your **true self**. In turn, you'll be happier. And happier people often eat healthier. Plus, once you identify your strongest chakra, it'll be easier to figure out more ways to best care for yourself through the many lifestyle decisions you'll make day to day.

Okay, so you may be wondering what a chakra is. Hang in there for the technical explanation. We'll make it quick.

Chakras are subtle energy centers in and around your body. Throughout time and across cultures, spiritual teachers and healers have known that chakras manage every facet of life: all things physical, psychological, and spiritual. They do this by regulating the two types of energy: physical, or visible, and subtle, or invisible. We define energy as "that stuff that makes up everything." That means your chakras are in charge of everything about you, the physical and the subtle.

We believe that most of reality, including much of your body, is fundamentally made of subtle energies. Actually, so do a lot of scientists. Developmental biologist Bruce Lipton penned his bestselling book *The Biology of Belief* about this exact concept. More than that, your subtle energies determine what occurs in your body. They actually serve as a blueprint upon which your physical cells organize and build. So if you make decisions that ensure your subtle energies are in good shape, your body and emotions will be too. In other words, if you support your chakras—the "brains" of your entire self—you create, bolster, and sustain your vitality.

Though every chakra is important, your true self, or soul, is embodied in one chakra more than the others. We'll talk more about that in chapter 1. What this means is that when you nurture your primary chakra, which requires consuming a specific set of foods and supplements, you'll find yourself automatically following a personalized eating program—one that will *work*. You can also use the knowledge about your primary, or most important, chakra to make all sorts of other lifestyle decisions, such as selecting the best forms of exercise or meditation. Though we'll emphasize your food-related choices in this book, we'll also provide chakra bonus tips to cover additional lifestyle categories, including grocery shopping and dining out. To make it fun, we'll help you uncover the special intuitive ability that lies in your strongest chakra and show you how to apply it to health decisions.

Excited yet?

Ultimately, our book boils down to this: We've all been told, "You are what you eat." Our motto flips that around: *What* you eat should be based on who you *really are.*

We're giving you more than a framework for eating with this book. We're offering a brand-new way to know yourself. Why *not* embrace your uniqueness and nurture your soul, as well as your body? No more comparing yourself to other people. No more worrying if your weight is slightly higher or lower than what it "should be." (PS: our plan will help you achieve the most harmonious weight for you, which means the pounds on the scale will align with whether you have enough energy for the important things—or not.) No more feeling guilty about making food and other lifestyle choices that differ from the latest fad or your loved ones' choices. You know what we're talking about, right?

You watch your partner follow a diet that's full of lean poultry and grains, but when you try to give up red meat or add more grains, you feel sluggish or lack energy. Or you go for the latest fad and remove all carbohydrates from your diet. And then—you can't focus! No more of that. This plan lets you customize eating based on your chakra type.

Instead of the typical seven-chakra layout you may be familiar with, we work with the twelve-chakra system Cyndi developed decades ago. A natural intuitive since childhood, she has always been able to perceive chakras, auric fields, and additional subtle energies and beings. Learning about the seven-chakra system when she was in her twenties confirmed what she intuitively perceived, but she could also see five additional distinct balls of light. She spent years investigating cross-cultural chakra systems and conducting her own research in order to identify and label these chakras. And now you get the benefit of her hard work! Using Cyndi's groundbreaking approach affords a deeper, more revealing, and more precise personality profiling of your energy, which in turn, instructs you how best to nurture your personal energetic makeup.

Okay, we'll stop. You might be gasping. We know that some of you are still insisting there are only seven chakras. So it's time to fill you in on a couple of skeletons in the chakra closet.

Most Westerners believe there are only seven chakras because, about a century ago, Sir John Woodroffe, under the pseudonym Arthur Avalon, wrote a book called *The Serpent Power*. His book became the source for most Western yogic chakra systems. Based on his work, nearly everyone decided that there could only be seven chakras.

However, even Woodroffe stated that the world's ancestors touted *many* chakra systems, with as few as two and as many as dozens of chakras. Plus, Woodroffe never actually said there were seven chakras. Rather, he offered up only six! Know that you can more precisely analyze your essential self when you have more, rather than fewer choices. You'll be glad we're this precise.

A QUICK TOUR OF THE BOOK

So you know what to expect in this book, here's a quick breakdown.

- *In part I,* you'll learn all about chakras and the twelve-chakra system. We'll also talk about what we mean by "health," "healing," and "harmonious weight," the three buzzwords in our tagline. You'll then take a quiz to figure out *your* major chakra type. In fact, you'll end up with a chakra ranking, a full portrait of your strongest to weakest chakras. You'll pay the most attention to the short description provided about your major chakra, but we'll also help you deal with any anomalies in your results.

For instance, what do you do if you have two strong chakras? We'll show you how to select which one to work with. What if you deeply relate to or desire to develop an aspect of a weaker chakra? You can still embrace it. Throughout the book, we'll weave together *all* the pertinent information about yourself. You'll be able to see a quick description of all the chakra types before jumping into part II.

- *In part II,* you'll find a write-up, or profile, for each major chakra type. You'll look up your major chakra and read all about yourself. Who doesn't like to read about themselves? Yup, strengths and weaknesses will be in there, but also information about your life purpose, intuitive gifts, main motivations, deepest fears, and that all-important main endocrine gland that you'll actually be "eating for." We'll then provide in-depth information about the foods and supplements that best support each chakra—especially *your major* chakra.

   We'll also give you a few extra tips about each chakra's specific health and wellness needs in areas including exercise, grocery shopping, and dining out. Then you'll focus on a few questions. These will help you clarify what data applies to you.

- *In part III,* you'll take everything you've learned about yourself to create a "chakra map," or plan. This is your customized food and supplement program. You'll use the knowledge you'll acquire from filling in these mapping sheets to develop a menu and a go-to grocery list. But you should consider other important nourishment factors as well, such as goals for exercise and stress reduction. We'll also show you how to utilize the insights you discovered in your chakra profile in part I and from the questions in part II. Say you want to eat certain foods from a secondary chakra type and skip some of them in your primary chakra. Well, you can! Or maybe you love the foods for your primary chakra type, but prefer the exercise and dining out tips for your second-strongest chakra. You can do that! You'll be ready to make concerted decisions that will fine-tune your diet and light up your life.

Are you ready to get to know yourself a bit better? We're excited you're on this journey: a step-by-step guide into your chakras—and your true self.

Part I

WHAT DO YOUR CHAKRAS SAY ABOUT YOU?

You're about to embark on an exciting journey: the discovery of *yourself*.

Do you ever think about your purpose, or wonder why you're here? Let us tell you. You are on this planet, at this time, to help lift our earth to a higher, brighter, and lighter place. And in order to help the world, you have to embrace and nurture your essential self.

You are worthy of a life that enables you to be unabashedly yourself at all times. And you deserve to be healthy in the way your natural self chooses to be healthy. On this journey, you'll learn about your chakras and why you want to eat and make healthy decisions based on them. Not sure how you'll learn so much about yourself? You'll take a quiz designed to help reveal your essential self. You'll love what you discover, just as you'll learn to love the self that emerges when you develop and follow the map of your soul.

1

ALL THINGS CHAKRA—
THE YOU INSIDE OF YOU

This is a wellness book based on energy—that isn't caloric. A book that holds information to help you reach your *harmonious* weight, not your *ideal* weight. Seems radical, right? Especially since the energetic system we're basing our food program on is all about chakras.

As we explained earlier, chakras are invisible energy centers that organize your entire being. Each plays a different role physically, psychologically, and spiritually. But not all chakras are created equal. As we'll explain, you have a main chakra. It's not just a key to your soul's destiny, but also to your health. If you nurture and cater to your strongest chakra, you'll nourish your entire self. You'll heal age-old issues and defy cultural judgments to achieve the weight that is best for *you*. Think of this new system as a shortcut to better health.

Here's our basic promise: we're devoted to assisting you in achieving health, healing, and a harmonious weight. Your way. In this chapter, we'll offer stories that show you what we mean and examples from others that illustrate how to accomplish your goals. We'll then break down the twelve chakras and give you some examples of the different chakric personality types. The first case studies will be about us. (You might learn a little more about us than you'd like!)

By the way, as you read through all this information about chakras, don't worry if you can't figure out what chakra type you are yet. The quiz in chapter 2 will help you determine your main chakra—and the nature of your soul.

TMI: HOW WE EAT FOR OUR TYPE
(For those of you older than Dana, more like Cyndi's age, TMI means "Too Much Information.")

We have created a one-word code describing each chakra type. This label is a quick way to summarize your core, soul-based personality. Since Cyndi is a strong first-chakra person, she is a Manifestor. Her center of gravity lies in her hip area and draws on the adrenals. We'll share what we know about Cyndi physically, psychologically, and spiritually simply because we know she's a Manifestor.

Physically, Cyndi is high-speed, if not a bit hyperactive. She runs until she collapses. Psychologically, she's all about security. That makes her vulnerable to negative emotions and fears about safety. It also makes her an impatient, "can-do" person. Spiritually, she makes intuitive decisions based on how they'll impact her body and material reality.

These first-chakra traits aren't good or bad. They don't make her better or worse than other people. This profile simply means that, to achieve her spiritual purpose, she *must* express these qualities. Otherwise, she's not going to get where she is destined to go.

This profile also means that she needs to support her first chakra more than the others. By making her food and supplement choices based on this chakra, and the specific endocrine gland associated with it, the adrenals, she'll automatically be at her best. Following the recommendations associated with her chakra type will create health, or a state of wholeness; healing, or the chance to repair the effects of choices not made in her best interest; and her harmonious weight, the weight that assures full-on passion and energy.

Cyndi is great at supporting her Manifestor self. She boosts her adrenals with her foodstuff choices. Since adrenals are stoked by lean protein choices, especially those that include the full panel of amino acids, she loads up on chicken and lean steak. Given the adrenals' propensity for burning up tons of energy, she takes extra mineral and vitamin supplementation, namely B vitamins, vitamin C, and zinc.

By making these food choices, Cyndi accomplishes more than fueling her physical self. As you'll learn, there are subtle energy benefits to various substances, as well as physical benefits. Proteins give strength. A Manifestor needs a lot of that! Minerals support the entire physical body, while B vitamins and zinc give an extra shot of energy and vitamin C keeps her immune system boosted so she can go, go, go.

While bolstering herself with the right diet, Cyndi also boosts her first chakra with supportive lifestyle choices. One highlight is that she doesn't meditate the same way several other chakra types do. Like other Manifestors, she doesn't even like to meditate!

First-chakra types don't sit. They don't close their eyes until they're ready for sleep. In other words, her mindfulness activities have to include movement. Toward that end, she runs her two big dogs at the dog park every morning in the dark. She can tune out the world while tuning into her body. By following this regimen—captured on her personal chakra map (you'll make yours in part III)—she's healthy as can be. Illnesses, if they do land in her body, don't last long. What may keep someone else down for a week will typically be flushed out of Cyndi within a day.

It took a little longer to repair old shame issues. For Cyndi, shame was kept in place because she was making unhealthy choices that didn't suit her personality. Her childhood issues had her weight tending toward heaviness as a way to deny the family shaming. Once she embraced who she was—and made the choices right for her chakra type, no matter what her family thought of her—her body found its natural, harmonious weight. These days, she's in great shape, at a weight that lets her flow from activity to activity, literally sprinting around the dog park. (She doesn't actually know how much she weighs. She figured out long ago that the number on the scale doesn't reflect well-being.)

Unlike Cyndi, Dana is a strong eighth chakra Mystic. It's a tough chakra center. If you're a Mystic, you can access all the chakras equally, which can be overwhelming. How can you nurture all your chakras at one time? You can't. The solution for Mystics is to select a chakra to focus on and mindfully attend to it. And that's what Dana does.

Dana's second chakra also tests up strong, so she employs a second-chakra approach to health. She selected this chakra because the emotional gifts in that abdomen-based chakra bring strength and power to her work with clients. Her choices make her a Creator, with her pivot point in the ovaries. Thus, Dana's health program looks quite different from Cyndi's.

For example, Dana is naturally nourished by whole grains and lighter forms of protein than those that Cyndi eats. While hyperactive Cyndi aims to eat three balanced meals a day plus snacks, Dana wants to eat—and craves foods—based on her feelings. When happy, she makes sustaining food choices. When not so happy, here come the cookies, or maybe nothing at all, because her appetite disappears. Because of this tendency, Dana's chakra map includes ways to coax her into eating healthy whether she's feeling up or down. For instance, she'll process a challenging feeling before she grocery shops, or she'll talk on the phone to a friend (probably Cyndi) while filling up her cart so as to keep her on track. (Otherwise, too many chocolate bars make it into the cart.) Her self-care includes the all-necessary processing of feelings, as well as time to innovate and create.

Adhering to her second-chakra self has released Dana from thinking it's wrong to have too many emotions. Understanding her own feelings has helped her realize which emotions actually aren't hers. A lot of Creators also tend to have empathic abilities. With that under control, now she can feel all her emotions and use them to create. On the slimmer side, Dana has learned to disregard the pointed comments from people who say, "You're too small; you should gain weight." All her creative energy keeps her healthy and thriving, and her Creator foodstuff program takes the fret out of decision-making.

Based on these descriptions, you can see how different Cyndi and Dana are from one another. While Cyndi is up early running two big dogs, namely Lucky and Honey, in the cold Minnesota weather, Dana is hunkered in bed feeling emotions. If she isn't happy, her poor little French bulldog, Sufi, may get robbed of her long morning walk. Not to worry, though; Sufi is in love with the neighbors and takes herself to their house to play when she doesn't get a good walk.

Are you more like Cyndi or Dana—or maybe Sufi? Sufi is a fourth chakra Relater, requiring lots of social time and friend connections. (Yes, animals have chakras too! You can use the quiz in chapter 2 to figure out your pet's main chakra if you want to. You just have to take the quiz thinking about them, not yourself.)

Don't worry if you're not like Cyndi, Dana, or Sufi. There are eight other chakra types, so you're bound to find your perfect fit.

EXAMPLES: HOW DO THE DIFFERENT CHAKRA TYPES EAT?

As you can see from our personal examples, each chakra type eats differently. For example, if you're a third chakra Thinker, your organ is the pancreas, and you'll tend toward hypoglycemia. Because of this, you'll want to eat frequently to balance and stabilize your blood sugar. Are you a sixth chakra Visualizer? You'll pay as much attention to what your food looks like as you will to what proteins and minerals it contains. If you're a seventh chakra Spiritualist, chances are you're rising early to spend your first hours sitting in a yoga position meditating, and only afterward will you eat. A Relater like little Sufi? Then you'll want to eat with others; food is more enjoyable when munched with company you love.

Of course, we are human, so we blur around the edges. Cyndi isn't only a first chakra Manifestor. She has a lot of sixth chakra Visualizer in her. In fact, she knew this about herself before she knew what a chakra was. As a child, she wouldn't eat food that touched other foods on the plate. Guess what? Decades later, she's still like that. To create her chakra plan, or map, she has inserted a lot of actions supportive of her sixth chakra. For instance, she puts her food on pink plates, her favorite color.

And Dana gets tired of dealing only with feelings. To compensate, she's mixed a few first-chakra ideas into her map; she is sure to eat enough protein and gets moving no matter what she feels. She is also nourished by tending to her Naturalist type and does this by choosing organic foods, as well as ensuring that she often gets out in nature.

As you can see, Cyndi and Dana have incorporated other important chakra-type traits and needs into their chakra map. You might want to do that too—or not. That's the cool thing about this program. You get to make it your own. You can even revisit it and switch up your plan if you're feeling like you want to develop another part of yourself because your map is customizable to you, whatever phase of life you're in.

WHY DOES THIS SYSTEM WORK?

There is one main reason that this chakra-based program works. It's energy.

Your body, thoughts, desires, cravings, and food—they're all made of energy. Absolutely everything boils down to one of two types of energy—physical or subtle.

Physical energy is measurable and is the topic of most diet, exercise, and self-care programs, as in counting your incoming and outgoing calories, for example. But when you focus too much on physical energy, you'll be prone to fall into cultural ideas that aren't ideal for you. Ideas like: Never eat before bedtime, only lazy people are overweight, food cheating is naughty, you're only as successful as your appearance, fat is bad. Just think of how many societal norms keep you from feeling normal and hold you hostage to what we call "the calorie checkbook idea":

Keep count and watch what you eat, or you'll be fat, ugly, and unacceptable.

Subtle energy, on the other hand, is like quantum, psychic, or spiritual energy. Our book focuses on subtle energy, which is the mainstay of your chakras. It's also the energy that, when balanced, leads to health, healing, and that "just right" weight for your particular lifestyle.

Chakras are an interwoven system of subtle energy centers that manage both physical and subtle energies. You can't see them because they are made of subtle energies, but they are in charge of what shows up in the physical reality. In fact, you could compare them to the behind-the-scene workers who move around the set pieces in between the acts of a live show. They do all the heavy lifting that makes your reality happen.

There are twelve basic chakras. Seven of them, the ones you may be familiar with, run along the spine. The other five originate outside of the body. Those are the ones that Cyndi could see when she was really young and that have become the basis of her world-famous twelve-chakra system.

Physically, each chakra links to an endocrine gland and also controls a different physical, psychological, and spiritual aspect of your being. That means every chakra runs the invisible *and* visible energies in its domain. So, here's the logic. If you want to improve your health, you have to focus on your chakras. But your health choices can be made even easier than that. If you tend to your strongest chakra, then optimum health can be yours!

WHY *EXACTLY* IS ONE CHAKRA STRONGER THAN THE OTHERS?

Okay, so it's important that you understand why you have a single most important chakra. This teaching doesn't only apply to making food and other health choices. Your most vital chakra can also give you clues about who you really are. That's because your soul, before you were born, encoded a certain chakra so you could fulfill your spiritual destiny. We'll walk you through this.

Imagine that your soul is floating around in the heavens before birth, wondering what it should become. The answer? An opera singer!

There is a single chakra most vital to singing. That's the fifth chakra, located in the throat area. The fifth chakra is about verbal expression. The next decision is easy. Your soul "lands" most heavily in the fifth chakra. Sure, you'll require the assistance of all the chakras to meet your goal, but if you take care of your main chakra, the rest will be cared for too. Nurture that fifth chakra and you'll not only be healthy, but might just become a world-class opera singer.

Is the soul intending to become a professional athlete? That person would nurture their first chakra, located in their hips. That's the chakra devoted to physicality and bodily movement. A wannabe academic or scholar? Bring that third chakra online, in devotion to mentality.

Since every chakra is related to a certain place within the body and a specific endocrine gland, each requires different supports to keep you healthy. Know your strongest (soul-based) chakra and you can make your health decisions accordingly.

The decisions you make based on your chakra/soul/true self will make you healthier in the most genuine sense of the word. But we know that you probably won't make *only* healthy decisions. As we've previously shared, health equates with wholeness. You're not only on this planet to work. Or to obsess about food. Or to be compulsively intent on any single part of your life. You are here to express all of you. The you who loves eating ice cream cones at the zoo. (Don't worry, we never say never.) The you who wants to write a book or build a bookcase or sail the wild ocean. The you who loves cuddling on the couch or running in the rain or eating pancakes on a Saturday morning. Supporting your most vital chakra creates energy for everything you're on this planet to experience.

Following a self-love foodstuff plan also enables healing, the process of releasing what doesn't fit you. Think of how many years you've been making so-called health decisions based on comparisons, or on issues related to culture, gender, professional standards, or what a friend suggests. Whatever you've done that doesn't align with you can lead to regrets. Actions taken just for others result in resentments. But every step taken to create your true self releases you from the regrets and resentments that get in your way.

Ultimately, you'll find that following your chakra map will lead to harmonious weight. In music, harmony occurs when individual notes join to make a pleasing whole. If your body turns into a temple for all parts of your true self, it will be pleased. You'll be pleased. We could care less if the number on the scale is "perfect," only that it is perfectly aligned with your real goal: to express all of you joyfully.

Recently, a friend of Cyndi's was insisting she couldn't be happy until she lost that last five pounds. "Nobody loses those last five (or ten or twenty) pounds if they don't need to," Cyndi told her. And that's the truth. Neither will people gain that five or ten pounds if their soul doesn't require them to. Let your soul lead. Then you'll be in perfect harmony.

QUICK REFLECTION

Take a moment to do a check-in. What do you believe is your goal or direction in life? Think about the activities you love. Are they physical or intellectual? Do you prefer spiritual solitude or spending time with family and friends? Ask yourself questions like these as you read through the next section, "What Are the Chakra Types?" and determine which chakra type you mainly identify with.

WHAT ARE THE CHAKRA TYPES?

Which of these quick portrayals best describes you? You don't have to decide yet; for now you can just dive into the process. You can also look at **Figure 1** as you read along and track the locations of the chakras.

MANIFESTOR. The first chakra, often called "the root," is anchored in the hips and Manifestors are all about movement and manifesting.

CREATOR. The second, or sacral, chakra resides in the abdomen. Creators focus on emotions and creativity.

THINKER. Located in the solar plexus is the third chakra. Third-chakra people are experts at "digesting" mental and intellectual energies.

RELATER. Ah, the beautiful fourth chakra, anchored in the heart. Little wonder that Relaters embrace all things related to love and relationship.

COMMUNICATOR. The fifth, or throat, chakra is pinpointed in the thyroid. Communicators are happiest when expressing, whether it be via speaking, reading, writing, or just plain ruminating.

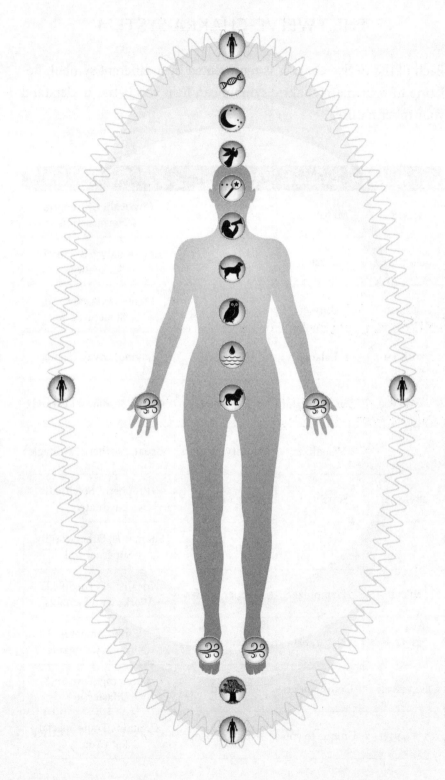

THE TWELVE-CHAKRA SYSTEM

Each of the twelve chakras is represented by a different symbol. Relating to your main chakric symbol can help you better understand your inner nature.

KEY

CHAKRA	LABEL	SYMBOL	MEANING
FIRST	Manifestor	Lion	Physicality, Strength, Determination
SECOND	Creator	Water	Emotionality, Creativity, Sensuality
THIRD	Thinker	Bird	Mentality, Analytical, Structured
FOURTH	Relater	Mammal	Loving, Loyal, Caring
FIFTH	Communicator	Expressor	Guide, Studious, Learned
SIXTH	Visualizer	Magnifying glass	Visual, Aesthetic, Strategic
SEVENTH	Spiritualist	Divine messenger	Prophetic, Spiritual, Meditative
EIGHTH	Mystic	Moon and stars	Shamanic, Otherworldly, Supernatural
NINTH	Harmonizer	Ladder of life	Idealistic, Principled, Works with Symbols
TENTH	Naturalist	Tree of life	Environmental, Outdoorsy, Organic
ELEVENTH	Commander	Wind	Directing, Forceful, Masterful
TWELFTH	Unique to you	Human form	Contains Traits Special to You

VISUALIZER. The sixth chakra, or third-eye center, is found in the pituitary. Within this space, we formulate insights, strategies, psychic pictures, and even imaginative fantasies.

SPIRITUALIST. The seventh, or crown, chakra is linked to the pineal gland. Connected to all things spiritual, it marks the Spiritualist, who is focused on higher concepts and truths.

Now we get to the out-of-body chakras. Even though these chakras aren't located in the physical body, they are tied to our physicality via specific organs.

MYSTIC. The eighth chakra, though positioned just above the head, is connected to the thymus gland in the chest. Through the eighth chakra, Mystics home in on the metaphysical dimensions of reality.

HARMONIZER. The ninth chakra is found about a foot and a half above the head, and locks into the diaphragm. It carries the key codes for a soul. Idealists at heart, Harmonizers love nothing better than to bring unification, whether to a group or a cause.

NATURALIST. About a foot and a half underneath the feet, the tenth chakra bonds us to Nature, but also to our personal heritage. Through the lymphatic organ of the bone marrow, the Naturalist serves the natural world.

COMMANDER. Surrounding your body, but more concentrated around the hands and feet, is the eleventh chakra. This energy center actually appears more like an energy field linked to the endocrine-related functions of the connective tissue and muscles. Commanders have the ability to control both natural and supernatural forces. Think changing the weather and casting spells.

UNIQUELY YOU. Let's pause. Reader: meet your twelfth chakra. Twelfth chakra: meet your special person. Your twelfth chakra looks like a giant egg-shaped field that surrounds all aspects of you. It actually reflects the attributes that are highly special about you. In fact, it holds the secret key to unlocking an intuitive gift that no one else has, making it a fascinating source of individuation and healing. We'll dedicate an entire chapter to helping you unlock your twelfth chakra's extraordinary traits, not because it will help you decide what to eat or not eat, but rather because that knowledge will grant you a power that will bolster your destiny. After all, isn't that what all of this is for anyway, to help you live as your truest self?

Do you have a sense of which chakra type best suits you? You'll get an even clearer picture in the next chapter.

2

WHAT'S YOUR CHAKRA TYPE?
TAKE THE QUIZ!

As we've determined, the chakra that most fundamentally substantiates your health and spiritual purpose needs special attention and specific care. All other chakras should also be healthy and functioning, but are less important in the overall picture of your life.

To tend to your most vital chakra—we'll call it your chakra type—you have to know which one it is. Don't be surprised if you have more than one strong type, though; it's pretty common. And if you're confused about that, relax—we'll guide you through what to do if that's the case. But in the end, we'll want you to concentrate primarily on one chakra.

Now, it's time to learn more about yourself through the chakra quiz.

Quiz: Your Strongest Chakras

While there are lots of tests and techniques for figuring out healthy eating habits and preferred fitness routines, this quiz is special. Why? Because it aims to help you identify your *energetic personality*. By taking this quiz, you'll identify your strongest chakra/s, and that knowledge will become the base for your personalized chakra map, something you'll accomplish in Part III.

Ready to find out your type? Let's do this!

Directions: Circle your replies to the following statements, deciding whether you agree or don't agree. We'll use a scale of 0 to 5. Zero means "I disagree completely," while 5 means "I agree completely."

If you feel unsure or confused about a question, just go with your gut. You'll score the quiz after you take it.

1. My eating is more out of control when I'm concerned about money.
   0 1 2 3 4 5

2. It's difficult for me to fall asleep if I feel emotional or upset.
   0 1 2 3 4 5

3. A good meditation will help clear my mind so I can focus on tasks and be more productive.
   0 1 2 3 4 5

4. I enjoy my meals more when they are shared with family and friends.
   0 1 2 3 4 5

5. I enjoy exercise more when listening to music or podcasts, watching television, or receiving instruction from a trainer.
0 1 2 3 4 5

6. I feel best when I make time to dress well and feel good about how I look overall.
0 1 2 3 4 5

7. I love to wear clothing that showcases my inner spiritual essence.
0 1 2 3 4 5

8. I enjoy my sleep the most when I am visited in my dreams by deceased loved ones or other beings who come in love.
0 1 2 3 4 5

9. When meditating, I prefer to access ideas and energies that could change the world for the better.
0 1 2 3 4 5

10. I sleep best when I am tucked into organic sheets and am wearing natural (or no) clothing.
0 1 2 3 4 5

11. I look forward to going to sleep so that I might dream about the potential gifts or superpowers I possess.
0 1 2 3 4 5

12. I like to be active throughout my day, and I feel frustrated if I have to sit still for too long.
0 1 2 3 4 5

13. When I'm emotional, I make unhealthy food choices.
0   1   2   3   4   5

14. I find it easiest to exercise when I have a set time in my schedule for it.
0   1   2   3   4   5

15. I sleep better when I am sleeping beside someone (or with a pet).
0   1   2   3   4   5

16. Reading books, listening to music, journaling, or talking about what's bothering me helps me de-stress.
0   1   2   3   4   5

17. My favorite meals are ones that are beautiful to look at in addition to being delicious.
0   1   2   3   4   5

18. I prefer to use my intuition along with spiritual guidance to determine what to eat.
0   1   2   3   4   5

19. When I'm stressed, calling on helper beings from other realms brings me peace.
0   1   2   3   4   5

20. My stress eases when I know I'm helping the planet or contributing to a meaningful cause.
0   1   2   3   4   5

21. I prefer exercise that gets me outdoors.
0   1   2   3   4   5

22. I look forward to sleeping so I can dream that I can fly and merge with the wind.

0   1   2   3   4   5

23. When I am sleepy, it's easy for me to put my head on the pillow and fall fast asleep, no matter where I am or what time it is.

0   1   2   3   4   5

24. In order to de-stress, I need to talk about and process my feelings.

0   1   2   3   4   5

25. I operate best when I live by a set schedule and routine.

0   1   2   3   4   5

26. I enjoy my life much more when I get to spend time with family, friends, and loved ones.

0   1   2   3   4   5

27. I fall asleep easiest when I am watching television or listening to music, an audiobook, or a podcast.

0   1   2   3   4   5

28. I feel my mood is impacted by the colors of the walls and art in my surroundings.

0   1   2   3   4   5

29. I feel a hunger for more spiritual knowledge and understanding of a Higher Power.

0   1   2   3   4   5

30. My curiosity gets piqued about subjects like aliens, angels, and magic.

0   1   2   3   4   5

31. Each year, I prioritize my time and money donations to organizations I believe in.
0   1   2   3   4   5

32. I feel best when I'm outside.
0   1   2   3   4   5

33. When working with another or in a group, I prefer to be in charge.
0   1   2   3   4   5

34. I get antsy when I have to sit still for too long.
0   1   2   3   4   5

35. I feel I am taking the best care of myself when I am doing activities that help me understand and process my feelings.
0   1   2   3   4   5

36. I feel satisfied when I am reading books, watching documentaries, or doing other activities that enrich my mind.
0   1   2   3   4   5

37. I am more motivated to work, exercise, or learn a new skill when I'm with a friend or someone I know.
0   1   2   3   4   5

38. When meditating, I prefer to have a voice guide me or music playing in the background.
0   1   2   3   4   5

39. How do I know I slept well? I wake up looking refreshed and revived.
0   1   2   3   4   5

40. I prefer to use my intuition or spiritual guidance to make decisions.

0   1   2   3   4   5

41. Most of my life I have felt like the odd one out; there is something different about me.

0   1   2   3   4   5

42. I won't take a job that doesn't serve a greater good or cause.

0   1   2   3   4   5

43. My favorite form of self-care is being outside, hiking, or somehow connecting to Nature.

0   1   2   3   4   5

44. When stressed, I tend to exert control over some external event, place, or person.

0   1   2   3   4   5

Scoring: On a piece of paper, add your scores for each of the eleven chakras that are listed in the chart "Adding Your Chakra Numbers." (We'll address Chakra Twelve in a later chapter.) For instance, under the Chakra One category, you'll add up the points scored in questions 1, 12, 23, and 34 and put them in the column "Total Scored." If you scored four points for question 1, four points for question 12, and two points each for questions 23 and 34, your total will be twelve points for that category.

Adding Your Chakra Numbers

CHAKRA AND TYPE	QUESTIONS	TOTAL SCORED
One/Manifestor	1____ + 12____ + 23____ + 34____	= ____
Two/Creator	2____ + 13____ + 24____ + 35____	= ____
Three/Thinker	3____ + 14____ + 25____ + 36____	= ____
Four/Relater	4____ + 15____ + 26____ + 37____	= ____
Five/Communicator	5____ + 16____ + 27____ + 38____	= ____
Six/Visualizer	6____ + 17____ + 28____ + 39____	= ____
Seven/Spiritualist	7____ + 18____ + 29____ + 40____	= ____
Eight/Mystic	8____ + 19____ + 30____ + 41____	= ____
Nine/Harmonizer	9____ + 20____ + 31____ + 42____	= ____
Ten/Naturalist	10____ + 21____ + 32____ + 43____	= ____
Eleven/Commander	11____ + 22____ + 33____ + 44____	= ____

Ranking Your Chakras

You'll be ranking the scores for each chakra in the Chakra Ranking Table. Next to each type, in the column labeled "Points Scored," write your total score from the section "Adding Your Chakra Numbers."

Your highest scores point to your strongest chakras. The lower a chakra's score, the lower its level of chakric vitality and importance. That means if you have a chakra that scored a twenty, the highest score a chakra can receive in this quiz, it is a more necessary chakra to your well-being and life destiny than a chakra that only scored a ten.

In the "Place" column in the "Chakra Ranking Table," rank your chakra types in order of high to low. If you have two or more chakras that received the same numerical score, these will have the same "place" number. For instance, if you scored twenty points for both Chakra One and Chakra Two, and these are your highest, you'll write "first place" next to both.

Continue with this exercise until you've accounted for every chakra.

Chakra Ranking Table

PLACE (FIRST, SECOND, THIRD, ETC.; CAN INCLUDE TIES)	POINTS SCORED	CHAKRA & TYPE
		One/Manifestor
		Two/Creator
		Three/Thinker
		Four/Relater
		Five/Communicator
		Six/Visualizer
		Seven/Spiritualist
		Eight/Mystic
		Nine/Harmonizer
		Ten /Naturalist
		Eleven /Commander

Debriefing

Now it's time to put everything together. Look at your highest chakra number/s. If you have only one—that's great. Then fill out the following lines.

My strongest chakras are: _____

_____

This makes me predominantly a _____ Chakra Type. (This answer can be plural.)

If you don't have a clear winner, that's okay. If your eighth chakra was your strongest, or amongst your strongest chakras, that's great too—except you'll have to do a little extra work. Read on to do that work. You can skip the next section if it doesn't apply.

IF YOU HAVE A STRONG EIGHTH CHAKRA AND OTHER SPECIAL CONSIDERATIONS

Here we go! What do you do if you're somewhat complicated? We'll show you how to pinpoint a single chakra.

1. Strong eighth chakra (Mystic). The eighth chakra Mystic is a confounding and wondrous person. You are the most complicated of chakra types because you are able to draw on every other chakra, and their intuitive gifts, to function. However, it's nearly impossible to create a food and health program if you try to tend to every chakra. Because of that, we want you to read the chakra descriptions that follow this section (under

"Chakra Types"). You'll then use the questions in the sidebar "Selecting a Chakra Type" to land on a main chakra. You'll still be given your own chapter in part II, because in addition to following the advice outlined in your chosen, non-eighth chakra, there will be additional tips related to your mystical greatness.

2. Lots of strong chakras. We still want you to focus on a single chakra. Answer the questions in the sidebar "Selecting a Chakra Type" to do that. You can also read through the related chakra-type descriptions in this chapter and part II to aid your process.

3. Lots of low chakra points. Most likely, you do have a strong chakra but it might not have fully developed. This can occur if you're in a life transition or perhaps weren't supported in being your true self during childhood. Pick your highest-scoring chakras and then read through the chakra-type descriptions in this chapter and part II. Then reflect on the questions in the sidebar in this chapter, "Selecting a Chakra Type," to determine your major chakra.

4. Equally high third (Thinker) and ninth (Harmonizer) chakra types. Want to know why we're homing in on these specific two chakras? Because they often go together. As you'll discover, Thinkers are highly analytical. Harmonizers focus on big thinking. If both are equally strong, it means you can focus on data and truth. We recommend that you eat for the Thinker type but integrate some of the Harmonizer ideas into your chakra map in part III. Our rationale is that it's more important biologically to nourish the Thinker organ, which is the pancreas, than the Harmonizer's, which is the diaphragm.

SELECTING A CHAKRA TYPE

It's helpful to decide which chakra to focus on when creating a chakra map. Reflect on these questions when you skim through the chakra-type descriptions in this chapter. If you need to, also skim through the applicable chakra-type personality descriptions in part II. This research will help you select a specific lead chakra.

Don't worry—you won't miss out on your other chakra preferences. You'll be able to mix and match applicable approaches for as many chakra types as you desire in part III.

Let's start by answering the following questions:

1. My most important life goal right now is:
2. The chakra that best relates to meeting that goal is:
3. After reading through the list of chakra-type labels, I believe my friends would insist I am this type:
4. My truest self would probably be best described by this label:
   (If you need help with this question, look at the list of labels we provide in the chakra chapters in part II. You'll find yourself in one of them!)
5. By adhering to this particular chakra type (_____),
   I can best serve my inner nature, my loved ones, and this world.

If you're still struggling with pinpointing a chakra type, we suggest you adhere to your response to question 4. Your answer to that question will be the broadest and most embracing of your truest self.

CHAKRA TYPES

Here they are! Brief descriptors of the eleven main chakra types. Read through just your own—or all of them—and then jump to part II.

Manifestor

Let's move! You make things happen—and quickly. Snap! Snap! All action. No stillness. You like to move, move, move, eat your three square meals a day (if you're not too busy), and meditate on the go. But don't worry: when it's time to sleep, you'll crash before you can say good night. Given that it's easy for you to make things happen—manifesting being your superpower—you have to watch out for your major weaknesses, which include being impatient with processes. You can become aggravated with people or systems that run at a different pace (usually slower) than yours. Lucky for you, you're able to draw on your physical empathy—the ability to sense what is occurring in other people's bodies—to help you understand others and tame that swift judgmentalism.

Creator

You're the feeler of the chakra spectrum. Every feeling is a color in the paint palette of your life, waiting to be waved about, expressed, and employed. You equate happiness with using all those feelings to create. Dance! Innovate! Draw! Write! You are all about making something new out of what already exists. Along the way, if you get to enjoy the sensual aspects of life, including touch and taste, you're in your best place.

When you're happy, exercise is easy and food tastes delicious. If your emotions are stirring, you'll be hard-pressed to enjoy anything, especially sleep. Unfortunately, you also absorb others' feelings. (Darn that emotional empathy!) Self-care necessitates owning your feelings and learning how to turn them into innovative sources of creativity.

Thinker

As a Thinker, you're in your head a lot. Busy in there, isn't it? You're always thinking, analyzing, and planning. You are the project manager, administrator, and organizer of the chakra zodiac. When you can create order out of chaos, you're blissful.

Lucky for you, you can draw on your mental empathy, or ability to understand others' thoughts and motivations, to make connections with data *and* people. Take a second and reflect. Don't others constantly insist that you have a great "gut instinct"? You do. Trust it. Just don't expect that others will trust it, and you'll refrain from one of your main weaknesses: being overly critical.

Food, exercise, and sleep happen on a schedule, or at least that's the way you prefer it. Overall, if you set and stay on a schedule, you'll minimize the stress in your life and accomplish all your daily tasks, including food-related activities.

Relater

You're the lover of the chakra types. Walk into a room full of people and you'll immediately know not just who likes who and who does not, but also who *needs* what in order to feel loved and whole. Have to choose a book from the library? You'll end up with the romantic one, no matter what's on the book cover.

As a walking, pulsing heart, your natural inclination is to help heal anyone who is even slightly out of sorts. Unfortunately, that tendency often leaves you not only caring for people but carrying them. The good news when it comes to food is you can use your relationship strengths to figure out how (not only *what*) to eat. For Relaters, meals are best with friends and family. In fact, everything is better with company, especially if you count yourself as good company.

Communicator

Reading, writing, and speaking. Those are your favorite activities. For you, the world is a verbal composition of sounds, tones, and statements. It's also a wide, wild space for one of your favorite habits: learning. In fact, if you're not learning, you're probably busy teaching someone something. Some of the acquired wisdom might come in through "normal" channels, such as books or the internet. Much of it, however, could be gained telepathically. After all, your main intuitive gift is clairaudience, or "clear hearing."

Because of your love of all things oral and auditory, food tastes best when accompanied by music or conversation. Exercise is more fun with a podcast piping through your headphones, and you sleep better when you drift off to background sounds.

Visualizer

You're the seer of the chakra universe. For you, joy is about beauty. Aesthetics are high on your list of necessities, and psychic visions or nightly dreams are quite commonplace.

Because of your visual nature, you might find yourself constantly imagining what could come to be. Wow! This visualization process often works to manifest your material world. Just be sure that you're focusing on others and the world around you as much as you focus on yourself.

Since you are visually focused, you love a pretty, plated meal. You can even change your mood by altering the appearance of the food *and* the plate.

As you'll learn, appearances can be more than skin deep. Exercise goes better when you're dressed for it—in matching or eclectic attire, of course. When you're stressed, if you can visualize the situation shifting, changing, resolving, it likely will.

Spiritualist

You're the seeker, the searcher, the one who is destined to embrace Oneness with your Higher Power. Prayer, meditation, contemplation: you've probably already figured out that these are three keys to a good life. In fact, you can most often be found in some form of spiritual connectivity rather than doing anything else.

Above all, you value your spirituality, as well as ethics such as honesty and justice. Be aware that your downfall can come from your ego, a totally self-focused aspect of the self. Too often, a Spiritualist's ego thinks it's always right and is always in perfect alignment with "God." If this is so for you, it might sometimes be hard for you to fully empathize with someone else's feelings.

Meditation connects you to a Higher Power, and your food choices must support your Zen vibe. Of course, you'll have to *do* something beyond deep prayer and meditation. What might unfold for you as you embrace nurturing yourself according to your chakra type? Your angel wings, of course.

Mystic

You are the shaman of the multiverse, the mystic who can easily converse with beings from other realms. All things otherworldly occupy your mind and your time. What exists that others can't see or hear? If you don't have the answer, you'll dive into the "mystery" to find out.

As a shaman, you can access and employ the soul gifts of every chakra. You can be clairvoyant (sixth chakra), prophetic (seventh chakra), physically empathic (first chakra), and so on. That can create trouble when you're making health care choices. What if your desire for meat, a first-chakra choice, clashes with the vegan value system inherent in your seventh chakra? That's why you must select a single chakra to focus on. What might be the healing outcome? Paradoxically, by limiting yourself to a single chakra, you connect to even more realms of light.

Harmonizer

Activism is in your blood. You weave together souls and spiritual principles in your own special way. In other words, "Kumbaya" could be your soul song. For you, life necessitates selecting a cause and focusing on it. Always, you lift the commonplace to a higher space, desiring nothing more than to create harmony where there has been disharmony and connectivity where there has been separateness.

That hypervigilance to harmony can make it hard for you to make healthy choices though. Your awareness of starving children can make it hard for you to enjoy your fancy dinner. But you can make wellness decisions that create a positive impact on the world and yourself. Exercise? No problem if it's a 5k walk or run that supports a cause you stand behind.

Naturalist

You're the nature lover. A bit of a tree-hugging, granola-loving, trail-hiking outdoor enthusiast. An all-organic fan and cosmic stargazer. For you, everything is about figuring out the best ways to unite with the natural world when making health and wellness decisions. At some point in your life, you've likely been called outdoorsy. You're all for being connected to the natural world, but be careful to not over-use your natural empathy. That's your ability to sense what is occurring in the environment or the beings in it, and that could be painful. For you, it's as soul crushing to sense what a tree feels when it's being felled as breaking your own arm.

In general, your food decisions will embrace the organic and chemical-free. In fact, all your health choices will be similar. Yup, you're the type found cuddled up in organic sheets while wearing cotton pajamas, or better yet, nothing.

Commander

Snap your finger and whoosh—wizardry occurs. Watch out, Harry Potter! You are the conjurer, the sorcerer, the wild commander of the chakra world. You might even be a Commander of the universe. Or at least your living room. Most of us aren't invited to play with natural and supernatural forces, at least consciously. But you are. So it's time to stop being a muggle. Your food, exercise choices, and meditation all will serve the same purpose, which is to strengthen your supernatural abilities. You may be a little weird, or perhaps a bit bossy, but that's okay. We want you to be weirder. In fact, the outcome of all this chakra work? To become the weirdest one of all—and love it!

Okay, you noticed. Chakra Twelve isn't here. As we told you, your Twelfth-chakra self is unique, so you'll figure out what it holds in chapter 15.

Once you have a sense of your strongest chakra, it's time to shift into part II.

Part II

THE CHAKRA TYPES—
THE UNIQUE YOU

We're going to cover a lot of ground in part II. It contains thirteen chapters in all. Twelve of them are devoted to the twelve chakras, one chapter each, and we'll give you an overview of how those are organized shortly. We know you're eager to explore the chapter devoted to your primary chakra type, but before you get there, it's important that we share some information that applies to all of them. So in the first chapter in part II, chapter 3, we'll cover both nutritional and energetic knowledge about the major categories of foods and nutrients that we'll be describing in the chakra chapters. The energetic knowledge is actually pretty darn interesting too. For instance, did you know that proteins always represent strength? That carbs are all about comfort? These subtle energy insights can make a difference when you're choosing what to eat. For instance, if you have to empower yourself for a meeting, don't select a carb. Go for a protein. You'll find loads of tips like that in chapter 3.

THE FLOW OF THE CHAKRA-TYPE CHAPTERS

Beginning with chapter 4, you'll find that the next eleven chapters are all organized in the same way. But the last chapter, about chakra twelve, is unique—just like your twelfth chakra. No matter what your primary chakra may be, in addition to reading its corresponding chapter, you'll want to be sure to read the chapter on the twelfth. It applies to everyone, and includes a process for uncovering your special self and spiritual gift.

To allow you to make the best use of the first eleven chakra-type chapters, we want you to be aware of the following details.

In the screened area at the beginning of each chapter, we'll tease the basics about your chakra type. We'll cover details about your essential purpose and the chakra's location, color, and associated affirmation.

After we outline these factors, we'll dive into your chakra personality traits. You'll learn about your intuitive gift and what really motivates you. We'll then highlight your strengths and weaknesses. After that, we'll discuss how to achieve and maintain a harmonious, healthy weight, as well as reasons you might be under- or overweight. We'll end the chakra-based personality section with a write-up about your chakra type's core endocrine gland and its functions. Basically, you'll make the most of your food-related and health care decisions with that gland in mind. We'll even provide you with a case study to help you relate. From that point, we'll launch into specific food recommendations.

After presenting a few quick tips dedicated to your chakra type, we'll explore healthy options for your proteins, fats, carbohydrates, vegetables and fruits, dairy, liquids, supplements, and to execute food tips, like how to make the perfect smoothie and items you'll want on your grocery list.

The next sections of each chapter are equally practical and food-related. We include a list of "Nopes": things that are best avoided by your chakra type. Then we provide real-life eating ideas like how to best do food prep, shop for groceries, and dine out—all according to your chakra type.

To wrap up each chapter, we'll present bonus material that covers exercise and movement suggestions, stress-reduction tips, mindfulness activities, and self-care recommendations. After all, when you're thinking about living the healthy life, remember: *living* is a verb! Included in this section will be at least one exercise to assist you in applying your intuitive ability to your life and food program. We'll end the chapter with a few reflective questions that will serve as the base of your customized chakra map, which you'll build when you get to part III.

It's a holistic—and whole new—way of looking at your health and well-being. Let's get started!

3

PRACTICAL TIPS ON FOODSTUFFS
FOR ALL CHAKRA TYPES

Think of this chapter as a guide to important information you'll need to know before you dig into the next twelve chapters, details that apply to all chakra types. We know. Details can be tedious and boring. But we promise ours are different! They're engaging, informative, and even fun. Fun because they will really help you benefit from the chapter(s) about your chakra type. As you read through this chapter, we recommend you make notes or highlight the ideas you'll want to remember.

FOODS TO AVOID AND THE NATURE
OF CRAVINGS

In general, you should avoid foods you are allergic or sensitive to. Unfortunately, many of us crave these foods. There are various reasons for this, including an energetic one.

A craving can occur if you associate a particular substance with an underlying emotional need. Usually, the related foodstuff *did* seemingly meet that need at one point in your life, most likely in childhood.

For example, imagine that your mother didn't hug you. Instead, when you cried she stuck a bottle of milk in your mouth. At a subconscious level, you learned to relate milk products with unconditional love. Years or decades later, you might still crave milk whenever you require a dose of love. Your soul, however, knows better. Your soul *knows* that milk doesn't cut it. Picking up that message from your soul, your immune system will attack either the sugar (lactose) or protein (casein) in milk. Now you have a full-blown allergy, or food sensitivity.

Another reason for cravings can be that you're missing something in your diet, or that you are reacting to a bodily instability. Chocolate cravings can happen because you're lacking magnesium. You may yearn for sugar if your blood sugar is low. Pay attention to your tendencies and see if you can track them to nutritional or lifestyle issues.

On the practical level, we encourage you to test for allergies or sensitivities with a medical doctor, allergist, naturopath, or nutritionist.

PROTEINS

All chakra types require healthy, lean proteins. For animal proteins, we recommend free-range poultry and grass-fed red meats, hormone- and antibiotic-free, as often as possible. Go free-range with eggs as well.

You don't have to be a meat eater, though. If you prefer a vegan or vegetarian diet, select approved proteins that contain the whole amino acid panel. You can also combine foods to create a full protein. Amino acids are what make up proteins, and you need nine of them at a time to qualify as a full protein. Vegan examples include quinoa, buckwheat, and hemp.

If you eat fish, try to purchase wild-caught—these have the lowest levels of mercury. And watch your balance of omega-3 and omega-6 fatty acids, which we discuss more in the next section.

FATS

There are three categories of good fat: polyunsaturated, saturated, and monounsaturated. Let's look at the differences.

In general, there are two types of pretty-much-always-good fats. One is polyunsaturated fat, which includes the omega-3s and omega-6s. In fact, your body can make all required fatty acids except for linoleic acid (LA), which is an omega-6, and alpha-linoleic acid (ALA), an omega-3. Both of these acids create the other necessary fatty acids. Fatty acids constructed from omega-6 are primarily found in animal sources, such as meat and egg yolk. Those formed by omega-3 are sourced from oily fish, such as salmon, mackerel, and herring.

On a deeper level, omega-3s support your adrenal glands' production and use of hormones, among other activities. Omega-6 fatty acids are great for your brain and muscles, but can create inflammation. Your takeaway? Avoid cooking with the omega-3s and omega-6s. These include sunflower, flax, corn, soybean, and safflower oils.

Okay, so maybe you can't cook with these fats, but you can eat foods containing them. Try fatty fish, sunflower seeds, walnuts, and flaxseeds. At times, you can cook with refined peanut, high-oleic sunflower, and high-oleic safflower oils. Do so seldom, however, as oils like peanut can have a lot of mold in them.

Some researchers suggest that we need a 4 to 1 ratio of omega-6 to omega-3 oils; others think you just plain need to get enough of both. We'll be recommending certain sources of omega-3s for certain chakra types, and omega-6s for others.

Let's move to saturated fats.

Saturated fats are mainly found in animal sources, like high-fat meats and dairy products. Tradition has given them a bad name, insisting that these fats clog the arteries and create other negative effects. Modern researchers aren't so sure. The best advice? Use these fats sparingly.

Because saturated fats withstand heat when cooking, they are beneficial when baking, broiling, sautéing, and frying. Just don't save and use them again because the molecules break down and the fats become rancid. Yuck. Saturated fats include butter, animal fat, coconut oil, coconut butter, cocoa butter, and palm and palm kernel oil.

Next we have the monounsaturated fats. These fats provide great energy, protect the heart, and assist with insulin sensitivity. Eating these can improve your blood cholesterol and decrease the risk of cardiovascular disease. They also help develop and maintain your cells. Foods rich in these fats include nuts, like cashews and almonds; veggie oils, such as olive and peanut; nut butters, such as almond, peanut, and cashew; and avocados and avocado oil. Check with a doctor to see what quantities of these you might want to consume per day.

Now we have a not-so-good category. These are on *every* chakra type's "Nopes" list. They are called trans fats or trans fatty acids.

There are two main sources of trans fats: natural and artificial. Natural trans fats are formulated in the guts of animals and foods made from these animals, such as cow milk and beef steaks. Small amounts of these trans fats are fine to eat. Then there are your artificial trans fats, which are constructed through an industrial process and found in processed foods. Think everything you like when you go for "cheat foods," like brownies, crackers, and more. Artificial trans fats are made by adding hydrogen to liquid veggie oils; this process makes them more solid and acts as a preservative. That's why they show up in so many packaged and frozen foods.

On a food label, trans fats are usually labeled "partially hydrogenated" oil. These types of oils, which include most corn and soy oils, are also always made from genetically modified organisms (GMOs) and can be drenched in dangerous herbicides. They make foods taste good, but increase chances of developing heart disease and stroke and can gear one up for diabetes. Steer clear of these fats, please.

CARBOHYDRATES

Carbs. We love them. We know that you do too. But not all carbs are created equal.

Years ago, everyone talked about carbs as organized into two categories: simple and complex. Well, carbs are more complicated than that and are now evaluated based on their glycemic index. Basically, this index is a way of ranking carbs that tells you how quickly they raise the level of glucose, a simple sugar, in your blood. In general, you want carbs to digest slowly, not quickly. Those that break down fast have a high glycemic index. Carbs that release glucose super slowly have a low glycemic index. Carbs with a middle-range breakdown have a medium glycemic index.

In general, minimize your high-glycemic carbs, eat a few medium, and go for the low. Here are some examples of each.

> **High-glycemic index carbs.** White flour products, all baked potatoes, white potatoes, instant oatmeal, short grain rice, corn, and sugars.
> **Medium-glycemic index carbs.** Orange juice, honey, sweet potatoes, yams, basmati rice, and multigrain, oat bran, and rye breads.
> **Low-glycemic index carbs.** Soy products, beans, chickpeas, lentils, brown rice, whole grain pastas, and grains, including bulgur pasta and steel cut oats.

Potatoes are tricky, so run your own research. Cooking methods actually impact the glycemic index. For example, sweet potatoes are generally low to medium on the glycemic index, but if baked for forty-five minutes, they turn into a high-glycemic carb. The answer? Boil them! White potatoes are also listed at the high end, unless you boil and eat them cold. Then they land in the middle range.

Another carb characteristic to use as a measurement is unrefined versus refined. You want to stick with unrefined carbs, which haven't been processed or are lightly processed. These include bran, barley, quinoa, whole grain cereals, and steel cut oats. Refined carbs will show up on your Nopes list and are super high glycemic. Stay away.

Now let's look at a few special carbs.

Sugar. A little note on sugar, which is a carb. (Okay, a long note.) Avoid it. Not just white sugar, but all of it. Even if it's all natural, from some exotic beautiful land, or brown sugar, which is actually white sugar with molasses, it's not good for you. Also say goodbye to corn sweetener and syrup, malt and invert sugar (a mixture of glucose and fructose obtained by the hydrolysis of sucrose), and anything ending in "-ose." Those sneaky -*oses*! They're whites playing dress-up in labels like dextrose, fructose, glucose, sucrose, and the like.

Don't eat the fakes either: sugar substitutes like aspartame, saccharin, neotame, and sucralose. They can make you shun healthy foods and have been linked to increases in various disease states—and sometimes weight *gain*, not loss. Instead, go for low-glycemic fruits or veggies.

The truth is we do crave and sometimes need a little something sweet. Experiment with healthier sugar substitutes for cooking or flavoring. Choices include dates or date sugar, monk fruit, or stevia. Some individuals can use pure maple syrup or honey, but we advise moderation in the use of these products because they can spike your blood sugar.

Gluten. Let's talk about another important carb issue: gluten. We know that eating gluten-free is a fad. Turns out, there is a good reason for this.

Gluten is a protein found in wheat, rye, barley, and certain other grains. People with celiac disease can't eat it at all. Those with mold or mycotoxin illness can start reacting negatively to gluten as well. But a lot of other people have gluten sensitivity, which can generate many of the same symptoms, such as diarrhea, bloating, gas, constipation, upset stomach, and a hangover-type feeling. Certain researchers believe that a lot of people are now reacting to gluten because of the residue from a chemical insecticide spray used on wheat in the United States that causes gluten intolerance. Specifically, this residue is called glyphosate.

No matter what you believe, it's smart to test your tolerance to gluten. You can simply abstain from all gluten products for two weeks and then reintroduce them, one at a time, to see if you react. Or work with a naturopath or functional medicine doctor to figure out your tolerance.

VEGGIES AND FRUITS

Technically, veggies and fruits are carbs, but they also occupy their own category. They provide lots of nutrients and fiber, are filling, and promote a healthy, harmonious weight. Like all carbs, vegetables and fruits can be measured by their high, medium, and low glycemic indexes. In general, the friendliest fruits and veggies are medium and low glycemic. A short list of these is as follows.

HIGH GLYCEMIC: Watermelon, dried dates, overripe bananas, and winter squash.

MEDIUM GLYCEMIC: Corn on the cob, figs, kiwi, bananas, pineapple, raisins, grapes, green peas, parsnips, mangoes, beets, and cooked carrots.

LOW GLYCEMIC: Green veggies, raw carrots, apples, grapefruit, oranges, peaches, pears, prunes, cauliflower, lettuce, mushrooms, onions, summer squash, zucchini, turnips, and peppers.

Want to increase your consumption of these health-loving veggies and fruits? Try these ideas:

- Use the rule of half. Load up half your plate with fruits and veggies for every meal.

- Steam and drizzle. Veggies are great steamed and drizzled with a spiced or seasoned healthy oil.

- Make smart substitutions. Order a side of broccoli, brussels sprouts, or asparagus at a restaurant instead of the baked potato. Switch out veggies for one of the eggs in your omelet.

- Dip it. Both veggies and fruits taste great with dips. Select healthy dips like probiotic sugar-free yogurt, hummus, or pesto.

- Make your own chips. Who doesn't love chips? Broil kale, carrot slices, apple, banana, or some other fruit or veggie on a pan sprinkled lightly with a healthy oil. Flavor as you desire for a healthy and quick snack. Using a dehydrator or air fryer makes this easy.

- Get six to eight. That's right. You want to get at least six to eight servings of veggies or fruits a day.

THE INS AND OUTS OF DAIRY

Some people can eat dairy and some can't. This statement is especially true in relation to cow dairy, which many of us were raised on. Having said that, dairy is considered healthy for many chakra types and individuals because it is loaded with saturated and unsaturated fats (depending on the type), calcium and other bone-building minerals, and nutrients. However, many people are sensitive to or allergic to certain types of dairy.

Many people lose their ability to digest the protein (or casein) and the lactose (or sugars) in cow dairy after childhood. Others are born allergic to cow dairy. Because of this, test your ability to digest dairy. Work with your doctor or nutritionist. Abstain from dairy (all types) completely and then slowly add it back in, checking for bloating, loss of energy, diarrhea, and other symptoms.

You may find you can tolerate goat, sheep, or even camel dairy. Some substitute soymilk or soy products for dairy. Soy can jack up estrogen and cause reactivity in many people, so test for reactions. Additional substitutes for cow dairy include almond or other nut milk products, coconut milk, pea milk, oat milk, and rice milk.

THE ENERGETICS OF VARIOUS FOODSTUFFS

One of the most important ways to decide what to eat and what to avoid involves an understanding of the subtle energetics of various types of foodstuffs. As you'll discover, carbs provide instant energy and comfort. If your best friend just moved away, you aren't going to crave a strengthening protein. You'll want a comforting carb. That's okay—just select a healthy one for your chakra type. But when you're headed to her going-away party? You might want to snack on a protein first, as you'll need the strength proteins offer.

The following outline of various types of foodstuffs and nutrients can key you in to the energies each substance provides.

Proteins for Power

Proteins grow and repair tissues. Energetically, they strengthen and empower, reducing your sense of being powerless or victimized by life's ups and downs. If you over-desire protein, you aren't in touch with your inner power or you mistrust your ability to cope with life's issues.

Fulfillment Through Fats

Packing more than twice the calories of proteins and carbs, fats store energy while insulating and protecting your organs. They also establish boundaries and protection, allowing you to feel fulfilled internally. Carrying too much fat around your middle—or anywhere else? You're overprotecting yourself, and are probably full of your own or others' shame. Fat can absorb shame, keeping you locked in a cycle of self-denigration or addictive tendencies. Empaths without healthy boundaries can pack on extra pounds that hold everyone else's toxic emotions. Can't keep on weight no matter what? You aren't embracing the wealth of love surrounding you.

The Comfort of Carbs

Providing sugar for energy, carbs deliver feelings of safety and lovability. They are all about comfort, contentment, and coziness. Cravings for carbs indicate you don't have a rich, internal source for self-satisfaction.

The Desires of Dairy

Dairy products leave us feeling gratified and satiated. When you want to feel taken care of, you may turn to dairy. Find new ways of caring for yourself and you won't need dairy to do the heavy lifting.

Waiting for Water

Your body is 70 percent water. Water molecules are crystalline in form, and can therefore be programmed by positive or negative philosophies. That means this nutrient transporter and cleansing agent carries your beliefs around in your body. If you avoid water, you probably hold a lot of destructive beliefs about yourself. Bless your water with life-enhancing affirmations and change all that.

Filling Up with Fiber

Fiber cleanses and removes waste. If you are chronically constipated or don't eat enough fiber, you might have a problem with releasing and letting go of anything from tangible goods to emotions and relationships. Do you have a lot of diarrhea or over-consume fiber? You might not be processing what you need to, from your emotions to awareness about yourself and the world.

Meaningful Minerals

These inorganic but necessary elements move life forward. There are many types and sources of the following minerals. You'll want to work with a nutritionist or naturopath to decide which suit you best.

Following are the energetic meanings of a few of your most necessary minerals:

CALCIUM. Calcium is required for healthy bones and teeth, but also to keep your muscles and brain moving. Energetically, it symbolizes the need for a healthy structure and framework upon which to build your life.

IRON. Iron carries oxygen and supports many chemical processes. It represents the ability to respond to stress and come out on top.

MAGNESIUM. Magnesium is responsible for more than 300 enzymatic reactions. Its jobs include relaxing your muscles and easing stress. It's also a secret weapon against illness. Required in every bodily process, magnesium also energetically represents your ability to allow your Higher Power into your everyday life.

POTASSIUM. This vital mineral is integral to muscle contractions, as well as heart and fluid functions. Metaphysically, potassium opens and shuts the doorway to the heavens. It is the counterpart to sodium, which grounds you in the here and now.

SODIUM. Salt is a busy mineral, maintaining normal blood pressure, supporting your nerves and muscles, and keeping your fluids balanced. Energetically, it provides the flavor of everyday joy. As the counterbalance to potassium, sodium allows you to reach for the heavens through the doorway that potassium has opened.

The Vitality of Vitamins

Vitamins are absolutely necessary for every bodily function. Each of these water- or fat-soluble nutrients reflects a quality you need to accept, process, and use. The following insights can assist you in making good choices:

VITAMIN A. Necessary for vision and tissue health. Supports your willingness to see truth.

B VITAMINS. Convert food into energy. Support your passions and goals.

VITAMIN C. A great antioxidant that invites meaningful connections and intimacy, as well as the clearing needed to support these relationships.

VITAMIN D. Strengthens the bones and reduces stress, even while it allows you to embrace all that occurs in your life.

VITAMIN E. Serves as an antioxidant and might protect from certain disease processes; can be anti-inflammatory. Represents your willingness to let go of old and others' energies.

VITAMIN K. Activates proteins and calcium for blood clotting. Allows you to accept your personal strength and control your negative thoughts and behaviors.

ONWARD TO YOUR TYPE

We know this is a lot of information. We also know you're chomping at the bit to dig into the specifics of your type. We're not going to hold you up any longer. Go ahead—flip to your chakra-type chapter and learn more about yourself!

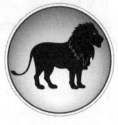

4

MANIFESTOR

Purpose: To Manifest
Your superpower is to manifest important stuff in physical form. That means you can achieve material success. You're about more than money and goods, though. You are a builder of materialized ideas and dreams.

Chakra Location: Hips
As a Manifestor, you're propelled by the first, or root, chakra. Anchored in the hips, it is located in the coccyx and runs energy through the adrenal endocrine glands. Keep your adrenals happy and you'll be your healthiest self.

Color: Red
If you were a color, you'd be red. Your fiery red energy invokes passion, energy, power, and determination. Like Hercules, you can get just about anything done.

Chakra Affirmation:
I am safe, strong, and passionate.

MANIFESTOR PERSONALITY TRAITS

The doer of the chakra zodiac, you are the most physical of all the types. You thrive by staying busy and taking action quickly. It's almost painful for you to sit still because you prefer to move, move, move.

That means you get things done. Once you make a decision, you're *on it.* No wasting time. Once you decide what to eat and not eat, you won't stray. But this isn't about discipline. It's about your true self, which does what's necessary to move you forward.

> **WORDS TO DESCRIBE YOUR MANIFESTOR SELF:**
> Doer. Driven. Busybody. Persistent. Motivated.
> Body-based. Kinesthetic. Achiever. Productive.

Your main intuitive gift is physical empathy. You can sense what is occurring in the environment around you. For example, imagine that you're sitting next to a friend who has knee pain. Soon you might start to think *your* knee is in pain. Basically, others' physical sensations can transfer straight into your body.

Now let's apply that aptitude to food.

You're at lunch with a cinnamon roll lover. Maybe you don't even like cinnamon rolls that much. But you find yourself ordering two and devouring them. What happened? You can catch cravings energetically. If this happens, you'll want to use the technique provided in the bonus section under "Mindfulness and Spiritual Practices" to clear out whatever isn't your own craving, desire, or physical issue. The empathic process under "Self-Care Rituals and Needs" will also help you make healthy decisions.

Your major motivator is success. You live for results. When you select a food program, establish success checkpoints. Tracking your progress and meeting your set goals will keep you on point.

Your hidden fear. You may fear facing early childhood or primal traumas, along with the unworthiness or lovability issues these traumas may have created.

Your greatest strength is your physicality. One of the reasons you're so physical is that the first chakra is the most body-based of all chakras. Red—the color of the first chakra—represents life energy. And you have lots of that. But there is even more super-greatness about you:

- Hard worker. You get it all done. When your lifestyle is balanced, your work ethic is admirable.

- Dependable. When you're in the zone, others can depend on you to do anything, from moving furniture to creating a dream business.

- Body enjoyment. You reap a lot of joy from the activities of your body, whether it's running that marathon or an all-night sex session with your partner.

- Decisive. Not only can you make a decision, but once you do—watch out. There's no stopping you.

Your greatest weakness is your impatience. Okay, we hate to break it to you, but just because you push tenaciously toward success, it doesn't mean you'll achieve your end goal overnight.

For you, the hardest part of a food program, or anything that requires diligence and time, is the need for patience. You'll get results, but maybe not tomorrow. So slow down and watch out for these other pitfalls:

- Distractedness. Staying overly busy means you may pay less attention to details, like stocking your fridge with healthy foods.

- Overindulgence. You work so hard that it can be tempting to say, "Sure, why not?" to that piece of cake.

- Workaholism. Enough said.

- Overcommitting. You have pie-in-the-sky dreams about all you can get done. Trying too hard can leave you fatigued and frustrated.

- Ignoring your health. Who doesn't overwork or overindulge when they're too busy?

- Passion. We've disguised this term. We mean sex. The genital organs are located in the first chakra. This means that sex is a great outlet for your stress. (We hear it burns calories too!) Unfortunately, you may confuse intimacy with sex. Sex does not constitute intimacy, and intimacy does not replace sex.

- Shame. We all fail. Or perceive that we do. Manifestors are particularly susceptible to thinking there is something wrong with them if they don't end up where they perceive they should be.

Achieving a harmonious weight. The key to a balanced weight is to release shame. Now, what's important to know about shame is that it isn't a feeling. It's actually a lie. It's the belief that there is something wrong with you. Sure, we all do stupid things. Forgiveness is key to healing yourself into a harmonious weight.

Typically, there are two main reasons for extra weight on a Manifestor. One is lack of safety. If you're insecure or being abused at any

---

CASE STUDY: BEN

Ben is a well-known builder in his hometown. A former college athlete, he enjoyed years on the football field—and an equivalent, larger-than-life appetite. As he put it, "Now that I'm in middle age, my middle-age spread just keeps spreading."

Ben simply couldn't keep his former habits from running his current life. He was used to late nights, huge meals, and a *push* approach to life. The latter included working fifteen-hour days, exercising only on the weekends, drinking a few beers every night, and forgetting to run just about any errand his wife or daughters requested.

Ben agreed to work with a nutritionist to figure out his best foods, and he also adopted several of our Manifestor approaches.

level, your body will hold weight as a buffer. The other involves stuffing your drive for success. You're great at helping others meet their goals, but you must ultimately strive for your own. Don't be embarrassed about wanting to become triumphant. Underweight? You're hiding your brilliance. Let it shine!

Your chakra endocrine gland is your adrenal glands; make all *your food choices with the adrenals in mind.* The adrenals—those two little organs atop the kidneys in the mid-back—are the stress organs of the body. One is on the right side of your spine, the other on the left.

They generate hormones, including adrenaline, hydrocortisone, and cortisol. Under pressure, these hormones pump you up. Afterward, your adrenals partner with other glands to calm you down. It's especially important that your cortisol be regulated, as it works with the brain to control mood, motivation, and fear. As a steroid hormone that is produced at different times of the day and night, optimally it reduces inflammation, regulates blood pressure, and assists with diges-

---

Even though he was reluctant, he agreed to eat balanced meals, starting with breakfast, always combining proteins, carbs, and fats. He packed snacks to carry with him when he was on the go and tried to eat dinner with his family every night. He also established a schedule that started with exercise early in the morning before anyone else in the family rose, and agreed to do the grocery shopping. That way, he began taking accountability for his food choices and learned about a lot of "newfangled foods," as he called them, like hemp and quinoa. He also embraced terms like "grass-fed" and "organic," even while complaining a bit about the cost. An item dropped from his shopping list? Beer. Instead, Ben started indulging in flavored water choices.

His greatest struggle was maintaining his new commitments. The idea of meditating made him laugh, as did making extensive

tion and the sleep-wake cycle. But stress can cause problems with the amount of cortisol the adrenals produce, as well as create hardships on nearly every bodily system. High levels of cortisol can be triggered by too much stress or a weak stress response, and cause you to get sick and gain weight. Too little cortisol? You could lose too much weight and become weak. Neither scenario is what you're looking for.

Have you heard the terms *adrenal fatigue* or *adrenal exhaustion*? They aren't official medical diagnoses; rather, they're labels that hint at a disconnect, or miscommunication, between the adrenals and the brain. An adrenal–brain disconnect can trigger symptoms that may include chronic fatigue, sleep and digestive problems, fuzzy brain, and cravings for the foods you're best off avoiding, like sugar, soft and squishy carbs, caffeinated and carbonated beverages, alcohol, and more.

Although they may not reflect a formal medical condition, burned out or overused adrenals are something you'll want to pay attention to as a Manifestor. For that reason, our food suggestions are heavily weighted toward building up or repairing the adrenals.

---

lists to organize his day. What helped him most was figuring out he was a physical empath. His wife pointed out that he often felt sick and complained about bodily pain. Using the exercises provided in this chapter, he began to separate other people's energies from his own and make behavioral and food choices that felt good to his body. His body stopped aching. He stopped eating whatever someone else was eating. He established better boundaries in all areas of his life, even sticking to a set bedtime.

And then, he made time for joy. He participated in dance lessons with his wife and started hiking with his girls. This newly developed and more peaceful approach left him less impatient with his family and employees. Yes, he lost weight, but more importantly, he became happier. And, occasionally, he still had a beer.

FOOD AND SUPPLEMENT PROGRAM
FOR THE MANIFESTOR

Ready for all the goods that will get you outfitted with a healthy eating plan? Here we go!

Quick Tips and Tricks for the Manifestor

These go-tos will help you create your healthiest body.

1. Eat for your adrenals. Think red!
2. Identify food sensitivities, allergies, and intolerances. You can work with a medical doctor, allergist, naturopath, nutritionist, or another specialist to figure out what to abstain from.
3. Find substitutes for your cravings. We most often crave what we shouldn't eat—our "Nope" foods. "Nopes" can trigger an allergy or sensitivity response, causing a rush of adrenaline and a quick feel-good moment. But the happy doesn't last, and your body pays the price.
4. Combine foods. To prevent adrenal-affected fatigue, eat a healthy fat, protein, and carbohydrate at each meal. Snacks too.
5. Eat whole, healthy foods. These will reduce inflammation, assist with blood sugar and hormonal balance, and provide clean energy so you can go, go, go.
6. Emphasize lean proteins and healthy fats.
7. Go for the greens! Lots of vegetables. Aim for six to eight servings a day.
8. Limit fruits, but if you eat them, consult the list in the next section, and exercise before or after to move the sugar through your system.
9. Eat at the right times of day for *you*. In general, most Manifestors don't like to eat until they're hungry. That tiny little preference can actually get in the way of a smart, adrenal-based rule of thumb. Because of the need to maintain blood

sugar—and cortisol balance—you do best when you eat break-fast, lunch, and dinner, plus snacks. If you don't, here come the cravings and the Nopes. Try these ideas:

- Wake hungry. That starts with eating an early dinner and then a small nighttime snack. When you awaken, eat breakfast. If you can't stomach it, move around for a while. Exercise. Get something done. Then eat. You've got to activate that blood sugar, or later you'll be snarfing not-nice foods. (We'll give you a great breakfast quinoa recipe in this chapter, so watch for it.)
- Eat lunch. Maybe on the early side.
- To curb that energy dip in the early afternoon, grab a snack. We like hummus and whole-grain crackers or veggies, probiotic (dairy or nondairy) yogurt and blue-berries, and maybe a mix of seeds and nuts.
- Eat dinner early! Try to dine between 5:00 p.m. and 6:00 p.m.
- Have a small evening snack. (Think small here so you wake up hungry.)

10. Hydrate. (Not with alcohol.)
11. Try fermented foods. They can assist your digestion.
12. You can have a small amount of sea salt. Most Manifestors can actually use a bit of salt.

Food Categories

It's all here! What to eat to help you manifest what you want to bring into your world.

PROTEINS: In the energetic world, proteins convey strength. What does a Manifestor want to be but strong—physically, emotionally, and spiritually? Go for proteins, but make sure they are of high quality.

Adrenals love proteins and prefer them mixed and matched with fats balanced with carbs. That way you can up your firepower without upping your blood sugar.

If you eat meat, go with beef. Make sure it's grass-fed, though; you don't need those extra hormones. You could also eat free-range chicken, bison, or turkey. A good fatty fish with lots of omega-3 fatty acids is good too. We're talking salmon, herring, or mackerel, maybe even a sardine or two if you have the stomach for it. Seek out the wild fish with the lowest levels of mercury.

What's the best way to prepare animal proteins? Lightly cook your meats. This keeps the amino acids intact. Remember to thoroughly cook chicken and pork, though. Raw meats like those can have nasties in them.

We almost hate to bring this up, given how old-fashioned this next suggestion might sound, but a Manifestor's adrenals love organ meats. An organ such as liver is flush with B vitamins, and those sweet Bs provide action energy. Plus, you could use the good cholesterol to help the adrenals make hormones.

You can most easily enjoy liver from beef or chickens, turkeys, ducks, or geese by making a pâté. Try our Liver Pâté recipe in this chapter.

Not a huge animal flesh eater but okay with animal products? Try ghee, which is basically clarified butter. It has been used in Ayurvedic medicine for centuries to aid the skin, hormones, and adrenals. You can find it in the grocery store or make your own. Here's how: Take a block of organic, grass-fed butter and put it in a dish in the oven at about 100 degrees F for an hour. Pour off the golden liquid at the top into a dish, discarding the white liquid at the bottom. Put the golden fluid in a glass jar and refrigerate. Use as you would regular butter.

Need to skip animal ingredients altogether? To create a full protein, put nuts, legumes, and seeds together, or go for hemp or quinoa, both of which are full proteins loaded with other nutrients. If you eat animal proteins, dairy and eggs can also supplement your diet. A lot of Manifestors do well with goat cheese, as it's pretty easy to digest.

MANIFESTOR'S LIVER PÂTÉ

For this recipe, use roughly a pound of frozen, grass-fed, organic liver. Defrost it, cut it into pieces, and then soak it in an acidic marinade. You can use lemon juice, lime juice, or your favorite vinegar. Sauté the liver along with a small onion, diced, in a couple of tablespoons of butter, ghee, or avocado oil until the meat is browned and the onions are tender.

Add to the pan a half cup of red wine or balsamic vinegar, and garlic, mustard, herbs, and lemon juice to taste. We recommend 2 to 4 cloves of garlic, a sprig of thyme, and 1 tablespoon of lemon juice. Simmer until the liquid is mostly evaporated.

Place the mixture in a food processor or blender. Depending on the consistency you want, you can blend it as is or add another tablespoon of butter or olive oil. Blend until creamy.

Set the pâté in a dish in the refrigerator until cool. Spread it on cucumbers, carrots, crackers, or gluten-free bread with veggies.

FATS: Healthy fats keep your adrenal hormones from spiking and provide consistent energy. In significant amounts, healthy fats can aid you in being relationally sensitive and personally self-accepting.

Fats should make up about 25 percent of your diet, if they are of the correct type.

For a Manifestor (and pretty much everyone else), trans fats are bad. So steer away from corn and soy oils.

Saturated fats used to have a bad name, but their advantage is that they can withstand heat when cooking. You can use them when baking, broiling, sautéing, and frying in moderate amounts. These fats can ramp up your chef skills: butter, animal fat, coconut oil, coconut butter, and palm and palm kernel oil.

Let's talk polyunsaturated fats, including omega-3s and omega-6s.

Omega-3s support your adrenals' production and use of hormones, among other activities. As we explained earlier, omega-6 fatty acids are great for your brain and muscles, but can create inflammation, which the Manifestor doesn't need more of. Your takeaway? Avoid *cooking* with sunflower, flax, corn, soybean, and safflower oil, but *do* eat foods with these fats. Sources include fatty fish, sunflower seeds, walnuts, and flaxseeds. At times you can cook with refined peanut, high-oleic sunflower, and high oleic safflower oils. But do so seldom, as oils such as peanut oil have a lot of mold.

The favorite Manifestor fatty fats? Monounsaturated. They provide great energy, protect the heart, and assist with insulin sensitivity. Get those bottles of olive and avocado oil. Avocado oil withstands heat better than olive oil, so lean toward cooking with that more often. And don't forget to snack once in a while on macadamia nuts and olives. (Macadamia nut pesto, anyone?)

Speaking of nuts, seeds and nuts contain a lot of nutrients and proteins, but did you know they also contain great fats? The following provide essential fatty acids, with a mix of the alpha-linolenic (omega-3s) and linoleic acids (omega-6s):

- Seeds, best consumed raw, include sesame, pumpkin, sunflower, and flax.
- Nuts, also best raw, include almonds, macadamia, coconut, walnuts, pecans, chestnuts, Brazil nuts, and cashews. If you eat nut butters, opt for dry roasted without added sugar.

CARBOHYDRATES: Manifestors love carbs because they invoke comfort, along with in-the-moment fast fuel. The best way to approach carbs as a Manifestor is to keep them whole.

Skip the refined carbs. The energy doesn't last long and it's taxing on your system. Complex carbs provide more energy that lasts longer.

Can you tolerate gluten? If so, whole wheat and rye are great choices. So are unpearled barley, unhulled millet, oatmeal, and the other grains that take a long time to move through the digestive system. If you are gluten-free, quinoa is a complete protein, as is amaranth, and you can cook with amaranth, pea, and buckwheat flour. Skip the white rice. Choose brown rice. Love potatoes? Go orange—think yams and sweet potatoes. If you like bread, get (or make) a loaf with lots of seeds (and no white flour). You could even bake a loaf with buckwheat flour and smother it in a seed and nut butter. Yum!

Beans like pinto, kidney, navy, and black, as well as lentils and chickpeas, are also good sources of low-glycemic, unrefined carbs. Hummus and bean dips are great snacks.

Need energy for the day? How about making a quick and healthy quinoa breakfast? It also works for dinner. Start by cooking two cups of quinoa. The package will tell you how, but we suggest cooking it in coconut or almond milk instead of water. In a glass mug, mix two cups of whatever milk you like, along with a half teaspoon of ground cinnamon. Take your cooked quinoa and pour the milk solution over it. Top with berries, nuts, and seeds. You can even stir in your favorite nut butter. To make this dish more dinner appropriate, cook in a bone, meat, or veggie broth and go for savory spices. Then you can add in roasted or sautéed veggies, such as kale, asparagus, broccoli, and carrots.

VEGETABLES AND FRUITS: Six to eight vegetable servings are recommended per day. We know that's a lot, but you can toss them in a smoothie along with some flax and hemp seeds and get a lot of vegetables in one go.

Best ones for a Manifestor? The brightly colored ones—think of the rainbow: green, orange, yellow, purple. We like the low-glycemic nature of asparagus, snow peas, zucchini, brussels sprouts, multicolored carrots, and dark leafy greens like kale, spinach, and collards. For the Manifestor, red veggies can be especially energizing. (Yup, time to load up on those beets, radishes, tomatoes, red peppers, and red cabbage.) If you're busy, buy already prepped or chopped veggies for the week.

Fruits aren't always the best for a Manifestor, as we've already said. Go for slow-digesting fruits like apples, cherries, mangoes, plums, pears, and papayas, and avoid the ones that might rile you up, like bananas. Test out your reactions to lemons, limes, and dark berries.

DAIRY: Goat milk and goat cheese are easy to digest. Probiotic yogurt (minus the sugar) can be helpful. A lot of Manifestors love dairy—it's one of the first-chakra favorites. Just make sure you aren't sensitive or allergic to it and check that it's free of hormones, antibiotics, and the like.

LIQUIDS: Water. Water. Water. As we mentioned in the Introduction to part II, water is crystalline in nature and can be programmed for various benefits. Want a little energy tip? Put your hand over your water and bless it with whatever qualities you require to give yourself that extra boost. A little green, herbal, or black tea can pick you up, but refrain from drinking too much caffeine, colas, and alcohol.

SUPPLEMENTS AND SPICES: Sea and Celtic salt are good additions for the Manifestor. Then splice in some extra immune-boosting C and D vitamins as well as your B vitamins to combat stress and provide energy. We love magnesium for Manifestors, although you should check with a professional for the best types. Magnesium L-Threonate is a great anti-anxiety mineral. We suggest taking it at night to reduce stress and induce the *zzzzz*'s. You can check out ashwagandha and licorice for balancing cortisol levels; however, avoid ashwagandha if you suffer from hyperthyroidism, as it can worsen your symptoms. Adrenal glandulars can help modulate adrenal moods. Tyrosine can be soothing, and curcumin is a great antioxidant. Cinnamon, too, is quite cleansing. Sprinkle it on your hot cereals or even sweet potatoes and yams. Want a crazy combination for a sweet treat? Try Dana's favorite way to eat a sweet potato: baked or boiled and topped with homemade cinnamon goat ghee and fresh rosemary. Sprinkle lightly with Himalayan sea salt and enjoy the magic.

The Nopes

Every type has an off-limits list. And guess what? These are often the very same foods that show up as cravings. Best to simply avoid them, and if you can't, work on the deeper issues beneath the craving. (Clue: they might have a lot to do with shame, one of your weaknesses.)

Here is a summary of what to avoid.

- The whites. You know this one. White sugar, white flour, white rice, and white potatoes. They are inflammatory and won't give you the kind of fire a Manifestor wants. Remember, no cane, brown, or "-oses"—sucrose, fructose, and the like.

- The fakes. Okay, so you can't have the "real deal" sugar, but while you're at it, stay away from the fakes too. We're talking aspartame, sucralose, and saccharin.

- Fried and fast food. Don't get fooled by fried and fast foods. They taste good, but are basically full of bad chemicals.

- Alcohol. We aren't saying you can never indulge, but alcohol has this odd effect on the adrenals. Initially, it lowers your adrenal function. Down goes the cortisol. You might sleep more easily—but you'll wake up in a few hours. If you overdo it, alcohol increases cortisol production, and that can throw your entire system out of whack.

- Soda. With sugars, fake sugars, caffeine, and all the other nasty components in them, can you see a benefit in drinking soda?

- Processed foods. Not real food, but food-*like* stuffs made through mechanical or chemical operations. Preservatives. Food dyes. Artificial flavors. Of course, you're not going to totally abstain. But limit, limit, limit.

- Caffeine—maybe. The jury is out. Some people thrive on caffeine, whether through tea or coffee, and some function much better without it. A lot of exhausted Manifestors keep themselves moving with caffeine, leading to more fatigue. We caution you against creating your red energy with caffeine. If you suspect you're dependent on caffeine to perk up your energy, abstain for a while and then use sparingly.

REAL-LIFE EATING TIPS

Since you're constantly on the go, we're going to give you some tips to make prepping, shopping, and dining out a breeze.

Food Prep

Manifestors don't have a lot of patience. But by simplifying cooking to mean the mixing of three ingredients and a fat, even you can find time to "cook."

To be jet-fire fast, prepare a few meals for the week. That way you won't grab the processed foods and starchy carbs or drink too much wine while you're cooking.

Want a few ideas about how to food combine?

Steak, brown rice, and broccoli all in the same pan, readied to be piping hot in a little avocado oil. You need very little prep time for this stir fry, and you can freeze the leftovers.

Pressure-cooked salmon and carrots. Place on a bed of spinach leaves, drizzle with avocado or olive oil, and you're done. Again, save the leftovers!

Snack time? If you aren't going to technically "cook," grab some nuts, or smear almond butter on an apple. You've mixed protein that's rich with good fats and a starchy fruit.

If you're too hurried to do the extras that go with a meal—like setting a table, lighting candles, or even using matching dishes and silverware—don't. Many meals can be eaten in entirety with only a fork or a spoon, depending on the food's consistency. With permission to shortcut, you'll figure it out.

Grocery Shopping

Do *not* grocery shop when you're hungry. You'll only stock up on Nopes. Also avoid the grocery when you're well stocked. You'll walk away with donuts and a chocolate bar or other craving-type foods.

Use your empathic style to sense how your body will react to a certain food. Just take a minute and feel into those veggies, whole grains, and protein selections. A food that leaves your body feeling happier, lighter, or more "up" is a good choice. The bad choices? They'll make you feel depressed, heavier, and more "down."

What really helps is to bring a grocery list to the store. However, list making and fast moving don't always mesh, so get a few ideas in your head and stick with them.

Okay, you hate lines. Order online and have the food delivered. Have to go to the store? Count the steps as you shop—walking is exercise, you know. You'll feel more productive.

Dining Out

Manifestors love to eat out, as long as there aren't long waits. Select restaurants that take reservations or move you through quickly. Ask for the bill to be brought out with the meal. We also recommend frequenting farm-to-table restaurants. Just about everything served there will be good for you.

BONUS MATERIAL—BEYOND FOOD

Beyond making conscious, first-chakra nourishment choices, you can support your health and wellness with activities that match your chakra type.

Exercise and Movement

To exercise for your adrenals, just *move*! Manifestors love to walk when others sit, jog when others walk, and run when others jog.

For balance, do exercise that gets you going as well as exercise that is more calming. Select a complete and intense aerobic exercise to perform twice a week or so. Examples include running, biking, brisk walking, downhill skiing, high-intensity interval training workouts, and other ambitious, full-body activities. Better yet—be competitive.

Most competitive athletes are Manifestors: go figure. Join a sports league, challenge a friend at racquetball, or get involved with a boot camp, and go for the win.

Balance your souped-up workouts with anaerobic exercises too. Mix them in a couple days each week. Practice patience with walking, doing martial arts or tai chi, weightlifting, and maybe even rock climbing if you like heights.

Manifestors are most successful at movement and exercise practices when they knock them out of the way first thing in the morning. While you may not want to keep a set schedule, it'll be helpful for you to at least formulate a plan in your mind for which exercise you're going to do each day. Once you decide to exercise, it's as good as done!

Mindfulness and Spiritual Practices

Ever try sitting in place and meditating? Even for ten minutes? Feels like an eternity, right? Manifestors don't sit still. So no more beating yourself up because you "can't meditate." Redefine meditation as being aware of what your mind is doing. Now add movement to it. Being mindful of your movements while cleaning the house, walking the dogs, cutting the grass, or scaling the side of the mountain can serve as meditation.

Martial arts and tai chi are spiritual and meditative practices. So are hot yoga and other fast-flow types of yoga. Kundalini yoga could be particularly beneficial, as it will draw your red life energy up into your spine, awakening more of your spiritual gifts.

Mindfulness in all activities is also a way to ensure you're not empathically absorbing other people's physical energy. Try the next exercise for clarity.

EXERCISE: "NOT MY ISSUE" MEDITATION FOR MANIFESTORS

If you suspect that you are holding another's physical issue or craving in your system, isolate in a quiet place but remain standing. Take a few deep breaths and set your hands on your hips. Keep them there while swiveling side to side. Then request that your soul release others' physical energies. Those energies will be returned to their source in a loving and kind way. Do this for a minute or two and then stop moving. Breathe deeply again. Then ask that your soul bring energy from the earth into your feet and legs. Allow that energy to rise up your spine and emit from the top of your head.

There. Much better.

Sleep and Relaxation

Let's be real. Of all the members of the chakra zodiac, you're the one who will drop when you're done. You don't even care about the nightlight or pajamas. When you're finished for the day, you'll pass out. Just don't get comfy with all the candles burning, and be safe for activities like late-night driving. Plan ahead; you don't want to run out of adrenaline in the middle of your drive.

Stress-busting and Prevention

Staying still can cause stress in a Manifestor. Get up. Take a break. If you're at work, go to the bathroom. Pause the video conference and do a quick jog in place. Get a stand-up desk or use a bouncy ball as a work chair. Ensure that you're moving during your day: walk from the back of the parking lot into the building; take the stairs when you can; or use the bathroom farthest from you. Also, twiddle. For real. Wiggle your toes, fingers, whatever it takes to burn off energy. The more you move, the more patient you'll be.

Then—as has already been suggested—have sex. Sex is a great outlet for a Manifestor. Of course, we don't mean indiscriminate sex. Healthy, consensual sex. Masturbation works too.

Self-Care Rituals and Needs

You'll probably have to force yourself to slow down and care for your bodily and emotional needs. Schedule self-care time and activities. Try bodywork. Massage. Acupuncture. Rolfing. Chiropractic care.

Therapy could be good too. Perhaps it's time to deal with those self-worth or shame-based issues. A good therapist can provide perspective in those areas. After all, are you sure those feelings of failure are deserved? Maybe it's a matter of looking at an event or relationship differently.

Since you're the chakra type least likely to take an actual vacation, we recommend you schedule action or adventure vacations. Go on a scuba diving or backpacking trip, or indulge your inner risk taker by learning a new sport.

Having a hard time deciding what might be a healthy activity for you? See the exercise "Making Decisions with Physical Empathy."

EXERCISE: MAKING DECISIONS WITH PHYSICAL EMPATHY

Your physical empathy becomes your best friend when you allow your body to guide your choices. The following steps can serve as a decision-making guide.

1. Think about a yes-or-no question and connect with your inner sage.
2. Breathe deeply while tuning in to your tailbone area.
3. While reflecting on your query, notice if the red energy starts to rise or fall. A "yes" flows upward, while a "no" descends downward. If the energy stays even, the choice is neither bad nor good.
4. If you get a "no" or a "maybe," test another option.

SELF-ASSESSMENT QUESTIONS

In order to build your chakra map in part III, you'll want to pick and choose from the concepts and tips provided in this chapter. Spend some time focusing on these questions, and take notes if you can.

1. What's one personal trait that you wish to fully embrace and build on?
2. What's a weakness that you now know to be watchful for?
3. Which foods from the recommended list are your favorites and should be included in your plan?

4. Which foods from the Nopes list do you need to take out of your current diet?
5. What are some possible substitutions for the Nope foods?
6. What do you fear could be the trip-up point, or downfall, of your new plan? Is there a professional or someone you know who could help you with that?
7. Take stock of your current pantry and food items. Are there any items you should toss out so as not to be tempted?
8. What recommended supplements do you already use, or want to start using, to support your health?
9. Which of the quick tips and real-life tips do you want to use?
10. What grocery shopping and dining habits can you change to help you follow your new plan?

And a few extra questions:

1. What are two forms of exercise mentioned for your type that appeal to you?
2. What one mindfulness or relaxation technique can you implement when stressed?
3. How about sleep? Is there a way you can improve it? Can you plan better to dedicate more time for nodding off?
4. Select a self-care ritual you know you'll do.
5. Is there another chakra that you would like to strengthen within yourself? If so, what foods or activities can you implement from that specific type to help bolster that chakra within you?

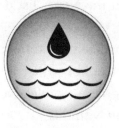

5

CREATOR

Purpose: To Create
Your soul is all about feelings, but you don't just feel them. You use them as a basis for the creation of a more abundant life, a more connected relationship, the ideal job, or the healthiest of bodies. Your emotional awareness, coupled with your compassion and empathy for others, makes you a powerhouse of creation and change.

Chakra Location: Abdomen
You're based in your second chakra, located in the lower abdomen. If you place one hand on your abdomen and the other on your lower back where your sacral vertebrae are, you're right on the spot. If you're a woman, your main endocrine gland is your ovaries. A man? The testes. Either way, your best-foods program will support your sexual gland.

Color: Orange
What color are you? Orange! Orange combines the gusto of red and the smarts of yellow to bring happiness, enthusiasm, and imagination. With a little encouragement, you can transform any feeling into joy.

Chakra Affirmation:
My emotions are good, and I am desirable.

CREATOR PERSONALITY TRAITS

You are an original. In fact, you *create* the original, fashioning anything, from a new idea to an inventive painting. Fundamentally, however, you assess the world (and food) through your emotions. Feel, feel, and then feel some more.

When you're expressing your feelings, magic happens. You become capable of heightened emotional self-awareness, and when you are aligned with self, you know what others are feeling and need. However, you'll successfully create your happiest body when most attuned to yourself and not others.

WORDS TO DESCRIBE YOUR CREATOR SELF:
Feeler. Empath. Emotional. Sensitive. Moody. Fluid.
Intense. Free spirit. Sensual. Wild.

Your main intuitive gift is emotional empathy. You experience your world through feelings. You feel your own, but also others' feelings. You are a feelings empath. Basically, you can absorb other people's emotions and reflect them back, like a feeling mirror.

It's a pretty intense gift, and it can make you everyone's best friend. They *know* you understand what they're going through. Heck, you'll likely sense another's emotional state or needs before *they* do! How many times have you sat with a friend and thought, *Well, they sure look happy for someone who's sad,* or *They sound awfully angry for being anxious.* However, if you're not adept at identifying the feelings that aren't your own, you may continue to feel another person's feelings. Not being able to separate your own from another's feelings causes trouble (even food-related trouble).

Picture this.

You're at dinner with a friend who is sad and lonely. You started out happy, but as the meal goes on, you start feeling heavy. Sort of like that soggy, buttery piece of bread. But wait! You already ate the entire basket of bread. What happened? Carbs provide comfort. Literally, you ate a ton of gooey bread to pacify those squelchy feelings that weren't even yours. Don't worry, though. We're going to show you how to prevent that.

Your major motivator is creating. You're an original. You rise and shine to fill this world with innovation in all forms. How do you alter the universe with your wild style? You transcend the traditional.

Your hidden fear is your own emotions. You may feel frightened of the strength and depth of your feelings. Work on embracing the power that understanding your emotions can bring you—and the truths your feelings can convey.

Your greatest strength is your emotionality. The second chakra is the holding place for feelings, sensuality, and beauty. Through your second chakra, you experience taste, touch, smell, texture, colors, and sounds. As a Creator, you are high on style. Think of your signature boots, fragrance, jewelry, article of clothing, special painting, or cool classic car. What is special to you makes you feel special.

Your emotions catapult you into a heightened sensuality, and those high feelings move a lot of energy. This also enables you to lift others to emotional highs. Your energy and empathic gift of connection can be addictive to others.

But your gifts can help you select more than your wardrobe or décor. Basically, foods that are good for you will activate a version of joy, such as happiness, bliss, satisfaction, comfort, or appreciation.

Your greatest weakness is your emotionalism. "Emotionality"—your greatest strength—is distinct from "emotionalism." Emotionality is the free flow of your own feelings and the support of another's feelings. Emotionalism occurs when we let our own or others' feelings take control. You know those too-big feelings that take over? They make demands like the following:

Anger: "I am *so* not okay with my needs or what I'm feeling. I'd better eat a donut."

Fear: "My friend's situation is so scary, I think I'll just lick the frosting off the chocolate cake."

Sadness: "I am drowning in sorrow. Who cares whose sorrow it is? Wine will fix it."

Disgust: "I'm so ashamed, I think I'll just eat all the candy bars in my kid's Halloween sack."

Guilt: "I feel so bad about hurting my friend's feelings that I'm going to punish myself with bad-for-me food. Is the pizza place delivering? Can I get extra cheese?"

Get the point? (We'll tell you what to do about those challenging feelings in a bit.)

Along with this emotionalism, you'll want to watch out for the following:

- Gluttony. Food delights the taste buds. As a highly sensual being, it's easy for you to overindulge.

- Sloth. Boredom isn't good for you. It's too easy to wallow in the bad feelings—and swallow all those snacks.

- Codependency. Another word for being *overly* empathic or taking care of others' feelings rather than your own.

- Creative mania. Wait. Didn't we say that creativity is your thing? Yes, but you shouldn't go crazy with the creative to the point where you don't eat or sleep. Remember to self-nurture.

- "Luxury" addictions. What are these? Shopping sprees, rich foods, gigantic muffins, expensive clothes or sofas, overeating—the sensual and sweet sorts of addictions that leave you feeling rich inside can also be your downfall.

Achieving a harmonious weight. What's the right weight for you? The one that makes you feel proud to have a body, that leads to the exploration of your sensuality. Tiny and quick, voluptuous, bulky? We don't care. Neither should you. If you have the energy to create and feel good, you're at the correct weight.

Guilt can be problematic in this chakric center, specifically if you feel guilty about your choices, feelings, and freedoms. Maybe you feel guilty for not donating, for donating too much, for saving, or for not saving enough. Guilt can be utilized to spark a quick check-in with your conscience about your personal sense of right and wrong. But for you, feeling guilt can often be troublesome. If you're struggling with guilt, see the exercise "Letting Go of Guilt."

Being overweight usually stems from repressed feelings or co-dependency. Ask yourself this key question to check for that issue: Are you weighted down with other people's emotions? Feeling guilty about something? Inability to gain weight can occur if you're failing to express creativity. Let it flow.

EXERCISE: LETTING GO OF GUILT

Guilt is an emotion that reveals a disalignment with our personal code of ethics. If you're feeling guilty, explore it, but leave behind the bad feelings. Here's how:

1. Take a deep breath. Let the breath fill up your abdomen with air and light.
2. Connect to your sense of guilt. Sit in it and with it. Keep breathing.
3. Focus on the experience that led to this guilty state. Then ask your inner sage or Higher Power what message the guilty

sensation is providing. How did you steer away from your personal ethics? Is there a corrective action you can take? In what way can you approve of your thoughts and behaviors? Follow the guidance you sense and then forgive yourself for any errors you made. Realize that others involved may or may not forgive you—but you can move on anyway.

4. Open your eyes and be free.

Your chakra endocrine gland is your ovaries or testes; you make all your food choices with these glands in mind. Physically, the ovaries and testes are charged with two vital tasks: providing half of the ingredients to form a new human being and producing sexual hormones. Both tasks mirror the Creator's major goals: innovating and enjoying life through feelings.

You'll need to constantly adjust your dietary plans to the cycles of your hormones and biological development. There are monthly cycles to consider, for both men and women, and also life cycles, which include pre-pubescence, puberty, maturity, pregnancy for women, pre-menopause/andropause, menopause/andropause, post-menopause/andropause. By moderating your food, you can modulate your hormones during all cycles, the same way that your cycles often guide your food choices.

Here's how your hormones and their cycles are tied to your food desires and needs. From an age perspective, a teenage male Creator produces a lot of testosterone, which provides tons of energy. He can tolerate less-nutritious food than can a fifty-five-year-old man in andropause with half the testosterone and a lot less energy to burn. (As an aside, the more testosterone, the greater the calorie burn. You can't eat as much when you're older!) Likewise, a young female Creator, her ovaries percolating along with plenty of estrogen and progesterone, can tolerate more dietary flux than a menopausal Creator, who has less of both hormones.

One unique challenge for the pre-menopausal and older female Creator is that estrogen is held in fat cells. When middle-aged and older women diet, this estrogen is released into their circulatory systems, throwing off their hormonal balances and potentially leading to depressed feelings, carb cravings, and weight gain. If a woman's estrogen falls too low, and her testosterone (made at this stage by the adrenals) remains relatively high, she might experience moustache growth, mood swings, and hair loss. If the estrogen is too high in comparison with the progesterone, the woman can experience bouts of anger and—of course—carb cravings.

It's easier to track the activities of the second-chakra hormones—and take them into account in relation to your emotions and food choices—when you have an understanding of the energetic meanings of the hormones. They are as follows:

- Estrogen: Feminine power, action, and protection

- Progesterone: Feminine calm, soothing, and comfort

- Testosterone: Masculine drive, success orientation, and power

CASE STUDY: FATIMA

Fatima was tired of crying about food. "I read through the chakra types," she shared, "and know I'm a Creator. The problem is, I'm only creative about ways to eat carbs."

Fatima was raised by a mother who passed out "the whites" instead of hugs and attention. Consequently, whenever she had an uncomfortable feeling, Fatima would reach for processed foods. When she felt unattractive? Bring on the hot fudge sauce, which she'd mix with a little bit of ice cream. When she was scared about asking for a promotion? Wasn't that what donuts were for? Helping a friend through a divorce? Pizza and wine nights, of course!

How can you apply these meanings? In the next section, we'll link protein, carbohydrates, and fats to your need for more estrogen-, progesterone-, and testosterone-subtle energies. We don't mean you're going to decide which food has the most estrogen versus progesterone. We mean you'll be able to select which of the three basic food categories to add or subtract based on the types of energy (feminine power, feminine calm, or masculine drive) you need. This sets you up for nutritional as well as emotional balance.

FOOD AND SUPPLEMENT PROGRAM FOR THE CREATOR

Ready for some specific food tips to create your healthiest self?

Quick Tips and Tricks for the Creator

Add these ideas to your list of how to create your own special eating plan.

Through our work, Fatima immediately benefited from learning how to separate her own from other people's feelings. She hadn't known how often she picked up others' emotions and assumed they were her own. When overwhelmed with these feelings, she nearly always regained composure by downing carbs.

She used our intuitive exercises and, with the help of a therapist, learned techniques for dealing with her own emotions. Whenever she felt a disturbing feeling, she would: Stop. Breathe. And trace it to its meaning and origins. With these processes underway, she became willing to make different food choices, substituting healthy carbs for unhealthy ones and eating more protein, which promotes power and strength. She also started doing food prep

1. Eat with your ovaries or testes in mind. Sounds weird, right? But you know what we mean—that's the place to focus.
2. Abstain from foods that cause sensitivities, allergies, and intolerances. They probably appear in the Nopes column. To help clear your system, work with a medical doctor, allergist, naturopath, or nutritionist.
3. Be aware of your vulnerabilities. Creators can be prone to various fungus, yeast, or bacterial issues. Trying to process others' emotions empathically, combined with a high-carb or unbalanced diet, can lead to digestive disorders. Check with your health care provider if you have intestinal troubles such as candidiasis, small intestinal bacterial overgrowth (SIBO), diverticulosis, Crohn's disease, or irritable bowel syndrome (IBS), or mold or biotoxin exposure.
4. Deal with microbial energies. The presence of healthy and unhealthy digestive microbes affects your food choices and vice versa. Because of this, it's helpful to understand the subtle

---

every Sunday with a supportive friend who kept her from snacking too much on her own inventive recipes.

She started feeling so good that she joined a yoga class to clear her creative channels. Fatima created a new self-image by making wild, brightly colored clothing choices. She then started volunteering for a local art organization and took sculpting lessons. She fell in love with sculpting, and that physical activity made her feel better about her own body.

Over time, Fatima not only began to love herself, but actually formed new friendships through the art community that left her too busy to overindulge in her former food choices. She also gained a list of friends to call whenever she felt so down that even a day-old donut might look delectable.

energy meanings of yeast and bacteria in particular. That way you can process the emotional energies, as well as shift your food choices.

- Bacteria can hold your own repressed feelings and emotions. So feel, feel, feel.
- Yeast and fungus can hold others' feelings. Release, release, release! Use the exercise "Not My Feeling Meditation for Creators" to accomplish this goal.

5. Manage your feelings to manage your food choices and vice versa. The enteric nervous system (ENS), also called the gut brain, is a significant part of your second chakra. It occupies most of your gastrointestinal system and is composed of thousands of neurons and glial cells. Glial cells regulate emotions. This system controls your digestive movements and hosts microbes, especially bacteria, that aid in digestion. The ENS also employs a two-way connection between the central nervous system (spine and brain) to affect your feelings, moods, and even consciousness, as well as various underlying disease states. For instance, if you don't eat healthy, you'll get in a bad mood. If you get in a bad mood, you won't eat in a very healthy way.

Want a tip on how to manage the mood part of your ENS? When you feel any of these feelings, respond accordingly:

- Anger: Set boundaries.
- Fear: Something is dangerous. Go backward, forward, or sideways. Just move.
- Sadness: I'm not feeling the love right now. I'll find a way to feel it.
- Disgust: Something is bad for me. I'll abstain from it.
- Guilt: I was off, so I'll become more ethical.
- Happiness: This is great! More of this, please.

Also, you can regulate choices and portion control by selecting foods after you've dealt with a major, too-big feeling. Don't choose your foods when you're all stirred up.

6. **Food combine.** Combine proteins, carbs, and fats for each meal or snack, but adjust the percentages based on hormones, if necessary. Here is your food-hormone formula.

   - Proteins provide strength and testosterone/male power. Too pumped up? Eat a little less protein. Acting wimpy? Grab more protein.
   - Carbs relate to comfort and progesterone/female calm. Lazy or tired? Don't overdo the carbs. Wired? Eat a few extra carbs.
   - Fats symbolize self-worth and bonding and estrogen/female power. Moody, angry, just in general feeling mean? Go for the fats. They'll bolster your relational compassionate tendencies. Self-hateful? Try fewer fats for the moment, work through a few issues of shame and guilt, and *then* go back to your fats.

7. Eat hormone-free foods and go whole and healthy. Do *not* add extra hormones to your diet, such as those found in meat and other animal products.

8. Stay hydrated.

9. Don't eat to escape other people's feelings. We've already said it and will again. You can absorb others' feelings, so free yourself from them and eat *only* for yourself.

10. Raise that fiber: super important for your intestines and digestive balance. You'll get less inflammation and better gut bacteria.

Food Categories

What's best to eat and not eat? Be creative and mix and match from what follows.

Proteins: It takes real power to feel emotions and generate creations, and proteins provide strength.

In general, avoid most red and all cured meats. Go for lean proteins. Enjoy a few ounces of fatty fish a week, such as mercury-free tuna and salmon; even shrimp, sardines, and crab can fit into your diet. Love grilled or baked poultry? Indulge in chicken and turkey. Eggs and nuts are full of selenium, a mineral we really like for you. It supports the ovaries and testes, and will keep you creating. You can also go for plant-based proteins, including beans and peas, quinoa, and buckwheat. Talk to your doctor about consuming soy, as the studies are mixed on the impact soy has on estrogen. If you get the green light, go for tofu, tempeh, miso, and edamame.

Men? Oysters do it for you. Like, help you "do it." They have zinc in them. Of course, you can supplement. Other good testes proteins include almonds, walnuts, and whey (if you're okay with dairy).

Want selenium-rich nuts and seeds? Brazil nuts are tops. So are sunflower seeds and cashews.

For a quick, any-time meal, try these muffin egg cups. They're nutritionally packed with all things good for your health.

MUFFIN EGG CUPS

Beat organic, hormone-free eggs in a bowl. Add in veggies and spices of your choice (see the sections below for specific ideas). We like tomatoes, spinach or chard, bell peppers, and herbs like thyme, rosemary, and oregano, plus salt and pepper. If it's your thing, add dairy (herbed goat cheese, perhaps) or nutritional yeast for a B_{12} punch. Bake at 350 F° for 20 minutes. You can eat as is, pop it on a bed of arugula and top with avocado, or use as a side for a sweet potato and pumpkin soup.

Fats: Okay. Fats may make you feel lovable but saturated fats, which are usually solid at room temperature, aren't great for your health. They are found in overly processed meats, animal products, and tropical oils, such as coconut and palm oil. Both saturated and trans fats can cause inflammation in the gut, but trans fats are worse, especially if they are artificial. You'll find the fake stuff in vegetable oils. Yuck. Avoid. You can tolerate the trans fats in dairy and meat if you keep portions minimal.

Instead, go for monounsaturated fats, such as olive or avocado oil. In fact, you can drizzle olive or avocado oil on just about anything that makes sense. Get creative.

Carbohydrates: Don't waste your carbs. We know your favorites: cake, muffins, pie, cookies. Every bite of those, however, reduces the number of healthy carbs you could indulge in instead.

Women with ovarian problems don't process carbs correctly. We're not saying you have that challenge, but you don't want to risk getting it. They aren't good for men either. Avoid refined, nutrient-deficient carbs. Far better, go for whole grains like brown rice, quinoa (it's a complete protein), buckwheat (also a complete protein), and whole oats and wheat, unless you're allergic to gluten. We've found that many second-chakra individuals can't eat gluten, especially if they have emotional issues from childhood. If your parents gave you gluten products instead of love and care, gluten can create an inflammatory response in your system. You'll reject the gluten as a means of turning down the "fake" love.

In general, go low-glycemic when you eat carbs, which turn into sugars more slowly in the body. But—a little dark chocolate once in a while never hurt a Creator. In fact, since we know you'll indulge every so often, make your own cacao-based treat with only three ingredients. (You'll use a little sweetener, so make sure it doesn't pump up your blood sugar.)

CACAO TREAT

Mix 1 cup melted coconut oil with 1 cup unsweetened (organic) cacao powder and 1 cup lakanto (monk fruit) syrup, or some stevia. Add in almonds; flax, chia, or sunflower seeds; or even a healthy, unsweetened protein powder of your choice. Form into balls and refrigerate. Voila! Bring these tasty snacks to events that might tempt you with less healthy foods.

Vegetables and Fruits: In general, you can eat as much fresh produce as you want. Fruit-wise, think strawberries, oranges, raspberries, blackberries, blueberries, passion fruit, apricots, papayas, mangoes, melons, and peaches. Go juicy and watery. Smoothies? They can have too many concentrated sugars, so be careful.

For veggies, think orange and red peppers, broccoli, yams, sweet potatoes, carrots, spinach, artichoke, and pumpkin. Mushrooms have a lot of your needed minerals and vitamins but are fungi, so go sparingly. Avoid them completely if you have any fungal issues like yeast or mold.

Dairy: If you aren't allergic to cow dairy, go for eggs and cow milk. Opt for organic and hormone-free. Many second-chakra types are sensitive to cow dairy, however, so have your health care provider test you. You'll bloat and feel horrible if you indulge and are sensitive, or you can get bumps like acne on your skin. There are a lot of good dairy milk substitutes, such as almond, rice, hemp, or coconut milk. Most Creators can eat probiotic yogurt and kefir. Just stay away from those with added sugar. Test yourself and see how you do with goat dairy. Goat milk, cheese, and goat ghee are products you may be able to tolerate.

Liquids: You already know water is good for you. It is! Can you down ten glasses a day to flush toxins? Herbal and green teas work too. Want a spritz of caffeine? Go for black tea. The jury is out on coffee; you'll know whether you can tolerate it or not. Stay away from fruit juice, sodas, and any beverage high in sugars. Bottled smoothies and cold-pressed juice only pretend to be good for you—they are sugary carbs. And if you're going to drink alcohol anyway, have a glass of red wine. Avoid the sugary or canned cocktail mixes.

Supplements and Spices: The second chakra loves minerals and vitamins. Both the ovaries and the testes especially like yeast-free selenium. (Strong sperm cells for men. Less ovarian cancer for women.) Vitamin C improves organ function and the flow of blood to the genital tissues and is anti-cancerous, while vitamin D supports you in multiple health areas, such as immunity and hormone production. Vitamin E can improve reproductive health. Vitamin B_{12} will regulate the flow of blood as well as neuron health, and niacin plays a major role in the production of sexual hormones.

Don't forget zinc! It helps you process your B vitamins, while ashwagandha keeps stress under control. Avoid ashwagandha if you have hyperthyroidism, though, as it can aggravate the condition. Also, talk to a practitioner about DHEA sulfate, which can boost testosterone and control estrogen.

Let's talk testes for a second. Decent "male tonics" include American ginseng and maca root. Omega-3 fatty acids can support the reproductive system, while saw palmetto berry is linked to a man's overall reproductive health. Yohimbe bark seems to enhance circulation in erectile tissues. Then again, some men check into D-aspartic acid, an amino acid that helps the testes make testosterone. Ever heard of tribulus? It's a plant known to enhance sexual desire, while fenugreek, an herb, seems to reduce the enzymes that convert testosterone into estrogen. A good amount of vitamin B_5 helps sperm too.

For women in particular, make sure you get enough vitamin A. You can find it in black currant oil, evening primrose oil, and (hold your nostrils first) cod liver oil. Yup. We recommend the burpless type. Stick it in the freezer and take it frozen to help reduce the burping.

Want to spice things up? Try garlic and onions. With breath mints. But you can also go herbal, using calendula, black cohosh, chamomile, and mint. Ever try paprika, cayenne, or horseradish? Raspberry leaf as an herb is also great for women in particular.

The Nopes

Putting it simply, your cravings go toward carbs. Love the medium- and high-glycemic ones? We'd really rather you not. Same for your enteric nervous system, sexual hormones, and organs. Your big Nopes follow.

- Emotional eating. Find your healthy place and choose out of joy.

- The whites. All Nopes!

- Fried, fast, and processed foods. This list includes french fries, donuts, and cake. And frosting. And chemicals, preservatives, and other yucky stuff.

- Too much alcohol. A little red wine is okay, but much else gives you sugar cravings. Avoid red wine too if you have fungus or mold issues.

- Soda. Not good.

- Caffeine—maybe. It's up to your system!

REAL-LIFE EATING TIPS

Now, how do you do your food in real life? We'll cover your ins and outs.

Food Prep

Create great meals! Come on—you are a Creator. Chefs are some of the most creative souls on this planet. Pleasing plating and a lovely array of colors make you happy.

Because you like to innovate, we recommend that you collect recipes and food magazines and try whatever you like. Learn to replace the not-so-good ingredients with healthier ones.

A lot of chakra types are best served by cooking ahead. Not you. You are a moment-to-moment, avant-garde wizard. Take time to cook. Create.

Want a few ideas?

- Baked yam atop grilled salmon (drizzled with olive oil) and a side of steamed, garlicky spinach sprinkled with paprika.

- Poached eggs on whole wheat (or gluten-free) toast with a bowl of raspberries in probiotic yogurt topped with coconut flakes.

Grocery Shopping

Most likely, you love to grocery shop, but only if the store is full of smiling clerks and bright and colorful fruit, and has a decent parking lot. As a Creator, you don't like depressed people or surroundings.

You also want to look good when you're shopping. You'll actually buy healthier food if you do. So wear a signature piece and bright colors. Refrain from sack-like clothing and those oversized old sweatshirts—you'll select tasty but unhealthy food. If you're feeling super low, don't go buy groceries. It's too tempting to load up on cookies and ice cream. Instead, stay home, and order in from a *healthy* takeout/delivery option.

Dining Out

Creators love to dine out. But if you are accompanied by a grumpy person, or if you're in the dumps, you won't make great food choices. Since your companions won't always be joyous—and neither will you—develop a short list of restaurants or cafés that pick you up.

BONUS MATERIAL—BEYOND FOOD

How else can you support your healthy lifestyle, based on your Creator personality? Read on to find out.

Exercise and Movement

A lot of Creators don't actually like to exercise. You'd rather get lost in the realms of feelings or manic creative moods. Exercise is good for you, though, especially if it plays up your sensuality, which is one of your strengths.

For you, full-body, skin-soft movements are the way to go. Swimming is a perfect option. Water is a primary second-chakra element and sure to soothe. Tai chi, Pilates, yoga, and dance are complete expressions of your soul.

As a Creator, choose a time of day to exercise when you're typically not overwhelmed with emotions or when you're ready to work out to blow off some feelings. For some, exercising first thing in the morning helps put a positive emotional spin on the day. For others, their lunch break is the ideal time to work off some steam. Or perhaps a slow-movement yoga class at night helps wring out all the emotions you've been plied with throughout the day. It's important that you schedule in your exercise and movement instead of waiting for inspiration to move your body.

Mindfulness and Spiritual Practices

Since you're all about emotions, let your spiritual practices provide you with the space to mindfully feel them. Try this for a quick way to learn that you *have* emotions, but don't have to *be* or act out your emotions.

EXERCISE: MINDFUL MANAGEMENT OF EMOTIONS

First, breathe into your second-chakra area, or abdomen. If you want to, put a hand there. Let a feeling surface and rise into your heart. Now ask yourself what feeling it is: anger, fear, sadness, disgust, guilt, or joy. Next, deliberately remain "at one" with this emotion. Let it be. Be in it. Then let yourself move with it. Any way you want. Dance, wave your hands, pretend you're a bird and flap your wings. In letting the emotion *be*, you develop emotional regulation.

For dealing with emotions that are not your own, perform the following exercise.

EXERCISE: "NOT MY FEELING" MEDITATION FOR CREATORS

As a feeling empath, it's easy for you to try processing another's emotions instead of your own. The following few steps will help you cleanse others' emotions and build energetic protection.

1. Sense where the emotional distress sits in your body.
2. Breathe into this area of discomfort and connect with spiritual

guidance, such as your soul or the Spirit, by whatever name you call it.

3. Request that the guidance flush the emotionally charged area with a bright and beautiful white light. This beam of light will wash others' emotions out of you and return them to their own soul, which can process them in a gentle and timely way.

4. Ask that this part of your subtle and physical body be filled with the exact shade of orange you require.

5. This same orange color will now blend with the white light and flow around your entire body. This orangey-white radiance fills any and all emotional holes and provides you safety and buffering.

6. Breathe deeply and return to your life.

Sleep and Relaxation

Creators find it hard to relax or fall asleep if they're emotionally down or wound up. And a bad night's sleep can cause a bad mood. Not a good cycle.

The solution is to address your problematic emotions before bedtime, or to give permission for your intuition to work on them while you're dreaming. The first task can be accomplished with a voice recorder or paper and pencil. Speak or write down every feeling. Shout or scribble and then cry, own, and feel. Then set all that aside. Burn the paper if you want.

If there are any intrusive emotions left—any that aren't a version of joy—ask that your soul obtain a diagnostic dream during the night. Keep a paper and pencil near your bedside to keep track of what occurs.

Guess what? Relaxing can be accomplished using the same process.

Stress-busting and Prevention

Want to prevent stress or deal with it constructively? Make something. We don't care what. A simple or a gourmet dinner. Invitations to host that dinner. A macramé shawl. A bookshelf. An organized closet. An online course or a nontoxic lotion. A company. A movement. A new kind of motor that burns trash for power. What to make is up to you. Do something creative every day to keep the doctor away.

Self-Care Rituals and Needs

This is a fun category for you. Your best self-care indulges your sensuality.

What are your most sensual pleasures? Getting or giving massages? Wearing one of those great hotel bathrobes while eating (a single piece of) dark chocolate? Inspired, all-day sex with your love? Crying at a rom-com or laughing at a comedy? Walking in the cold in your woolens while planning your next creative project? Come on! You can think of a longer list than this.

SELF-ASSESSMENT QUESTIONS

In order to build your chakra map in part III, you'll want to pick and choose from the concepts and tips provided in this chapter. Spend some time focusing on these questions, and take notes if you can.

1. What's one personal trait that you wish to fully embrace and build on?
2. What's a weakness that you now know to be watchful for?
3. Which foods from the recommended list are your favorites and should be included in your plan?
4. Which foods from the Nopes list do you need to take out of your current diet?
5. What are some possible substitutions for the Nope foods?
6. What do you fear could be the trip-up point, or downfall, of your new plan? Is there a professional or someone you know who could help you with that?
7. Take stock of your current pantry and food items. Are there any items you should toss out so as not to be tempted?
8. What recommended supplements do you already use, or want to start using, to support your health?

9. Which of the quick tips and real-life tips do you want to use?
10. What grocery shopping and dining habits can you change to help you follow your new plan?

And a few extra questions:

1. What are two forms of exercise mentioned for your type that appeal to you?
2. What one mindfulness or relaxation technique can you implement when stressed?
3. How about sleep? Is there a way you can improve it? Can you plan better to dedicate more time for nodding off?
4. Select a self-care ritual you know you'll do.
5. Is there another chakra that you would like to strengthen within yourself? If so, what foods or activities can you implement from that specific type to help bolster that chakra within you?

6

THINKER

Purpose: To Think
You're here to formulate ideas. Thinking is your jam. Your analyzing mind and ability to organize data are a part of your higher purpose.

Chakra Location: Solar Plexus
Your energy is anchored in your solar plexus, the area that stretches from the bottom of the rib cage to the belly button. Within this area lie most of the digestive organs, although your major endocrine gland is only one of them: the pancreas. This chakra also extends into the thoracic vertebrae behind the solar plexus region.

Color: Yellow
Sunshine and daffodils, even on a cloudy day. Ultimately, yellow conveys clarity—and you love clarity. Joy for you is understanding why something is the way it is. It makes sense, then, that the better you understand yourself, the more engaged your brain will be when making healthy food choices.

> **Chakra Affirmation:**
> I am powerful, intelligent, and successful.

THINKER PERSONALITY TRAITS

The brainiac of the chakra family, you love data. Even more, you delight in analyzing, categorizing, and applying all the information you know, even about food. How can your love affair with knowledge guide your perfect food program? No doubt that, as you read this, you'll be thinking about that.

We already know you can think. You also have other very strong traits, including the gift of mental empathy, or the ability to get into someone else's head. Read on and you'll learn all about it, as well as your major motivations, strengths, and weaknesses, and your special endocrine gland, the pancreas.

> **WORDS TO DESCRIBE YOUR THINKER SELF:**
> Brainiac. Data driven. Mentalist. Logical. Reasonable.
> Organized. Compulsive. Smarty-pants. Intellectual.

Your main intuitive gift is mental empathy. Simplistically put, you know what others are thinking. You even know what motivates them. This gift can sometimes twist you in knots though. It's not easy to handle knowing that someone is pretending to know something that they actually don't know anything about. (*There* is a tongue twister.)

Another term for your innate spiritual capabilities is "claircognizance," or "clear thinking." This means you can trust your gut when making decisions.

How does your gut-based intuition operate when making food choices? Well, it can work for or against you.

On the plus side: You follow through on your instinct for making a healthy choice. Go, you!

On the dark side: Your gut insists that you skip dessert. However (as your weaknesses will show), you don't like being judged. There you are, in a fancy restaurant, and everyone is ordering the tiramisu. So you go with pack mentality—and don't feel so well the next day.

We tell you all this to say: Trust. Your. Gut.

Your major motivator is positivity. You can do it! When you tell yourself this, guess what? You accomplish your goals. It's even easier to perform and make good choices if the peeps around you are optimistic. Nothing and no one gets in the way. However, while claircognizance can make you sensitive to other people's positivity, it'll also have you picking up on their negativity. Unless you develop rigorous boundaries, the negative will win—and you won't. Ugh. Use the exercise "Mental Empathy and Food Choices" to build positivity and home in on the correct food selections.

Your hidden fear is your own power. You know you're powerful, right? Stop playing small to make other people feel comfortable. Stop pretending you don't know all that you know. Embrace the dominating powerhouse you are.

Your greatest strength is your innate intelligence. You have the most inherent smarts in the chakra universe. (Now, don't go telling all the other chakra types that; you won't win a popularity contest that way.) Your love affair with facts and data, and their organization, makes you an amazing logician.

By approaching your food program with mental acuity, you'll formulate a structured plan and follow it. That's because you have these traits:

- You're logical. Reasoning can win over sugary temptations or the desire to skip a workout. Just talk to yourself. "If I eat this donut, I'll have

a sugar crash." "If I don't get to the gym, my energy will lag throughout the day."

- You're project-minded. You are the Structure King or Queen of the
  chakra types. Once you compose a plan, you'll commit to it unless an
  emergency arises.

- You're smart. You are intellectually and intuitively one smart cookie—
  which means you can talk yourself out of *eating* that unnecessary cookie.

You have lots of metaphysical assets too, which relate to the energetics of the organs associated with your third chakra. Every organ
fulfills both physical and subtle functions. Draw on the powers of
each organ to establish and follow a plan.

- Pancreas: Brings joy. In a nutshell, your pancreas assures you on-
  demand energy. Keep it healthy and you'll enjoy an even blood sugar
  level and an equally even temperament.

- Liver: Accomplishes goals. Cleans and purifies your blood, aids in digestion, and provides the power needed to accomplish any and all ob-
  jectives.

- Gallbladder: Achieves visions. Aids in digesting certain fats and vitamins. Energetically, fats represent richness, and vitamins serve the
  esoteric purposes covered in the introduction to part II. Gallbladder
  energy helps you process the concepts, principles, and ideas required
  to embody your life visions.

- Spleen: Focus. Your spleen is a very busy little organ. It fights certain microbes and assists your overall immune system. It also keeps
  your blood cells healthy. Energetically, the spleen helps assimilate the
  thoughts and ideas you gather through life, narrowing your focus.

- Stomach: Differentiation. Here, you break down food, fiber, and water.
  But you're also mixing thoughts and ideas, sorting what to believe in
  and not. Confused? Your stomach energy can aid you in separating
  others' views from your own.

- Small intestine: Process, process, process! All those good nutrients, along with the unneeded foodstuffs, get handled here. Keep your philosophies positive and you'll be happier.

Your greatest weakness is your vulnerability to negativity and judgment of others. Want great health? A Thinker *must* make decisions based on accurate and correct ideas and assumptions. This statement applies to beliefs about yourself and the external world.

Let's say you don't believe you deserve to be healthy. Your actions will automatically follow that belief. You might reach for the unhealthy carbs, which energetically represent connection, to give yourself a quick pick-me-up. Up goes your blood sugar—for a short time—before it plummets, as does your mood (and health).

Inaccurate thoughts can also come from the outside world. Imagine you've been taught you're supposed to eat three square meals a day. That style of eating doesn't work well for a Thinker type. Your pancreas thrives on being stoked many times a day. Base your health plan on others' ideas and you'll find yourself with swinging emotions and erratic health.

Because you can't control others, you need to keep your inner psyche positive. The third chakra is the home of beliefs and thoughts, many of which you procured in childhood, before you could assess their accuracy. Chances are, you've got some dumpster-diving, wrong, hurtful, harmful ones in there. These can cause poor self-confidence. And when these dysfunctional beliefs are running the show, you don't feel like exercising, so you won't. You won't stick to your bedtime plan either. Sure, you'll chastise yourself for sitting around and eating caramel popcorn (delicious!) or drinking beer, but you won't stop doing it.

As a Thinker, it's important to be aware of—and change—the six major negative beliefs that might be haunting you. Utilize the listed antidotes instead, either as affirmations or as a focus during meditation.

- I am unworthy to *I am worthy*
- I don't deserve to *I am deserving*
- I am bad to *I am good*
- I am powerless to *I am powerful*
- I have no value to *I am valuable*
- I am not lovable to *I am lovable*

Then watch for these traits:

- Perfectionism. If you become too precise, you can get overly careful about your wellness plan and drive yourself or others crazy, causing stress. Want to lose weight? You could cut so many calories you start to disappear.

- Excuse-making. You are so good at mentalizing that you can come up with seemingly justified reasons for putting off your wellness activities.

- Over-analyzing. What's the point of figuring out *everything*? Sweetness is often to be found in mystery and wonder.

- False pleasures. It's easy to convince yourself that you enjoy an activity when you don't. Be honest with yourself about what you truly enjoy versus what you feel you should do.

- Boundary issues. Sigh. It's easy to become too rigid or, conversely, too lax. Either way, the main problem is a lack of self-trust. Figure out your truth and your boundaries will follow.

Achieving a harmonious weight. You love fitting into your typically tailored clothes, unless you have that "let's slop around today" thing going. Your optimum weight? It will remain fairly even—if you follow your fine-tuned food and life plan. If your schedule gets out of control, your weight will likely fluctuate. Think it's too high? You are people-pleasing too much, not following your own sense of destiny. This can lead to feelings of anger and resentment, which can be a Thinker's downfall. If you're feeling angry, think about a boundary you can implement or an action you can take to help you feel empowered. Feeling resentful? Talk with a therapist or counselor and learn healthy ways to express your desires and opinions along with how to say, "No!" Underweight? You're overworking. Take a break. Or a lot of them.

Your chakra endocrine gland is your pancreas; you make all *your food choices with this gland in mind.* As we've shared, your third chakra, found in the solar plexus, encompasses nearly all the digestive glands. Most vital is your pancreas, the endocrine center of that particular chakra. The pancreas lies across the stomach region and is responsible for making insulin.

One of your pancreas's main relationships is with the stomach. After the stomach breaks down food, the pancreas creates insulin, a hormone that helps use or store certain types of sugars. The brain of the third chakra, your pancreas, assures that you have lots of energy for tackling life. If any of your third-chakra organs are working improperly, however, your digestion will be disturbed, and you won't get nutrients out of your food.

Nutrition, along with water and fiber, fuels every aspect of your life. If you aren't properly absorbing your foodstuffs, you'll feel lackluster and, eventually, exhausted and sick. Then again, if you are overeating, you'll become bloated, heavy, and potentially ill. Either way, it will be hard to organize your life, make decisions, and think clearly.

In particular, an unhealthy or untended pancreas can lead to digestive disturbances, diabetes, hyper- or hypoglycemia (high or low blood sugar), and even kidney or heart disease. Other third-chakra issues include problems with the stomach, liver, spleen, gallbladder, esophagus, and small intestine. If you already have one or more of these challenges, don't feel discouraged. By making decisions based on your Thinker style and creating a structured life plan, you can turn your health around and experience joy.

From an energetic point of view, the third chakra addresses more than the digestion of food. What's happening physically in the hotbed of your digestive system is also occurring mentally. That's right! While your third-chakra organs are busy ingesting, digesting, and assimilating nutrients, they are doing the same with ideas. Front and center in that chakra, your pancreas is figuring how to best use this data to "sweeten" your life.

FOOD AND SUPPLEMENT PROGRAM FOR THE THINKER

Now for the good stuff—food and other food-related recommendations.

Quick Tips and Tricks for the Thinker

Make these concepts your own and make your body happy.

1. Eat for your pancreas. Keep it happy and you'll be extra healthy.
2. Figure out your food allergies and sensitivities. We recommend working with a physician, allergist, nutritionist, or someone of equal knowledge.
3. Think through those cravings. Most of the time, we crave what we're sensitive to, which are usually the foods on our Nopes list. Those Nopes shoot up blood sugar, which makes us feel positive—temporarily. Then down goes the blood sugar. And here comes the negativity.
4. Time your eating. As a Thinker, you must eat with regularity because you're prone to blood sugar fluctuations. But the old three square meals a day? That won't work. You'll flourish by grazing, or eating several small meals a day. If you don't have time for a full mini-meal, you'll want to have some healthy snacks on hand to keep the "hangry" at bay. When you do eat, food combining is your friend. Each mini-meal should be a

combination of a low-glycemic carbohydrate, a low-fat protein, and a healthy fat. After all, a Thinker loves logical balance.

5. Go for whole and healthy foods. These will reduce inflammation, assist with blood sugar and hormonal balance, and keep you positive.

6. But stay away from high-fat foods and simple sugars. These can raise your triglyceride levels and put too much fat in your bloodstream. Same with processed meat and too much red meat.

7. *Stop!* Stop overthinking. Stop going for that candy bar. Stop spiraling in negativity. In general, you'll eat your worst when you're overthinking. Go figure, right? If you're stuck in a negative belief spiral, you'll crave high-glycemic carbohydrates. Push through by carrying around packets of nuts or small high-protein food bars.

8. Think it through energetically. Consider your reasons for eating. Cravings are a sign that something is out of balance. If your liver is angry, you may reach for crunchy junk food. If

CASE STUDY: DESTINY

"I eat really well until . . . I slip," shared Destiny, rubbing her hands together nervously. "Then I get the munchies and I can't stop eating. I hate myself when I do it. And the negative self-talk is out of control!"

Destiny struggled with a typical Thinker challenge: she could stay on track with a food and health plan until she got overwhelmed with dark thoughts, which was often. As a Thinker, she was intuitively vulnerable to her own or others' negativity.

Because she's a mental empath, many of Destiny's internal criticisms didn't originate within, but were thoughts she absorbed from others. Hearing this, Destiny flashed into a *eureka!* moment. "You mean, I'm okay the way I am?"

your gallbladder is rageful, you'll go for bad fats. Are you over-working? For sure, your life will be "under-sweet." Your pancreas might demand a candy bar. Push the pause button and think it through.

9. Consider adding one to two tablespoons of medium-chain triglycerides (MCTs) to your diet every day. We'll cover what those are in the Fats section later in this chapter.

10. Water is your best friend. But stuck Thinkers will reach for coffee, caffeine, beer, and the bubblies, as in bubbly soda pop. Don't.

11. Watch the crunchies. Lots of times, your cravings are for crunchies, which give you an outlet for anger and frustration. Deal with your anger first and you won't even need the popcorn, granola bars, and other crunchy, not-good-for-you foods.

Food Categories

What foods do you want to pay attention to—and not? Let's check them out.

Agreeing to grow her self-positivity, Destiny was then willing to establish a clear and clean structure to achieve health and well-being. For instance, she started grocery shopping at exactly 2:00 p.m. on Sundays and performed her food prep right afterward. To loosen herself up a bit and activate her creative juices, she listened to her favorite jazz musicians while creating a week's worth of meals. She also packed quick, easy munchies so she wouldn't be tempted to cheat with buttered popcorn—her favorite snack—while working. Her favorite healthy snack now? Crunchy celery with almond butter.

Destiny found she stayed on track most easily when she followed a set meal, snack, and bedtime schedule. When she traveled, she learned to pack easy foods to help herself stay on that

Proteins: In general, a Thinker's diet must include healthy proteins, like lean meats and poultry, or tofu if you're into soy-based food. Don't overdo the steaks, though. To give you some ideas, try indulging in turkey, chicken, duck, and goose. Add in some lamb, bison, veal, or pork. Seafood is also a good bet. Opt for prawns, shrimp, crab, lobster, scallops, oysters, and clams if you do shellfish. Eggs are also a good source of protein. Why do you need lean proteins? The pancreas is a protein expert. The protease enzymes made by the pancreas perform most of the protein digestion in the stomach and small intestine. Eat too much high-fat protein and you'll increase the need for these pancreatic enzymes, causing more strain on the pancreas.

A high-protein diet can also decrease your desire for carbs. So make sure you're eating enough of them. Carbs are full of minerals and vitamins, without which the pancreas would overwork. (We know you know what overwork is, perfectionistic Thinker. Don't do that to your poor little pancreas.)

Let's talk about diets that throw you into ketosis, like the Paleo diet. These diets are high in protein and fat and low in carbs, and help you lose weight. They also make the pancreas cook up more glucagon to release the energy stored in fat cells. As the fat cells break down, they give off a byproduct called ketones. In turn, these reduce your appetite—but they also strain your pancreas and other organs. Skip the ketosis diets unless working with a physician. Instead, balance

---

schedule. But she said what really helped her out was the tip we gave her about bringing her pillow with her. She swore it helped her sleep when she was stressed.

Destiny learned to evaluate her thoughts, and she would stop herself when she found herself thinking negatively about herself or a situation. She used positive affirmations to help herself flip the negative thoughts around quickly. Before long she reported that she was able to stop the destructive thoughts before they started.

your proteins with healthy carbs. Choose healthy, lean proteins, and, once in a while, indulge in an omega-3 rich fish. Legumes are great also, as are nuts and seeds, but be sparing with them.

Fats: We're going to start with a fat Nope. No fried foods. Nope, Nope, *Nope.* The more fat you eat, the harder your pancreas has to work.

Although it's important to be careful with fats for your sweet little pancreas, don't completely avoid them. About 25 percent of your diet should be fats. Go for oils like olive and avocado, but in moderation. Medium-chain triglycerides (MCTs), such as those derived from palm and coconut oil, can boost your mineral absorption, especially if your pancreas is a bit challenged. You can also ingest some healthy fats by occasionally eating fatty fish, nuts, and seeds.

An especially healthy and easy dinner? Pick a carb—okay, we'll pick it for you, since you haven't read that section yet. Brown rice. Stir-fry it with coconut oil, chopped veggies, coconut aminos, and tofu or chicken. Then drizzle with organic peanut oil, soy sauce, or more coconut oil. (There's gluten-free tamari sauce too.) Even better, add some pineapple as a topping. The pancreas loves the enzyme bromelain found in pineapple. And a few coconut shavings never hurt anyone.

Carbohydrates: In general, you'll want to jump into the next section, Vegetables and Fruits, and eat a lot of those. That's the best place to get your carbs. But adding in whole grains will help limit your cholesterol intake and increase your fiber. Be sure to select grains that haven't been stripped of their fibrous components, like the husk, germ, and bran.

Best to divide your grains like this:

- Low glycemic load carbs: Include bran cereals, beans, whole wheat tortillas, barley, oat bran, whole-grain pumpernickel and sourdough.

- Medium glycemic load carbs: Small portions of pearled barley, brown rice, oatmeal, bulgur, rye bread, and whole-grain breads and pastas.

Besides pleasing your pancreas, these choices will make your gall-bladder happy. (Ever had a gallstone? You don't want one.) You'll also lower your chances of having high triglycerides, a leading cause of pancreatic problems.

Beans and lentils are also great. Although they are stand-ins for proteins, they are also low-glycemic carbs. Good-bye potato chips, even if they're made out of veggies or yams, as you shouldn't be mixing that many fats in with your carbs. Instead, make up little snacks you can eat on the go, or as substitute meals. Try this: almond butter and celery, or cucumber and tahini. Better yet, make some hummus as a dip for carrots and jicama.

Vegetables and Fruits: The pancreas loves broccoli and other cruciferous vegetables. Ever tried cauliflower roasted in coconut oil? It's good. Trust us. The great thing about cruciferous veggies is that they contain compounds that eliminate toxins. Spinach and other greens provide lots of B vitamins, and lemons release necessary enzymes from the pancreas. Carrots are low glycemic, as are tomatoes. Look for yellow veggies and fruits like corn, squash, beans, and oranges (okay, they're orange, not yellow, but close enough). For fruits, select those that contain a lot of digestive enzymes, such as papaya and pineapple. Berries are great too! Perhaps you might put bananas on the list. Though they are relatively high glycemic, they provide instant energy and are certainly better than a candy bar.

Okay, we'll give you a cheat food. Craving sugar? Sweets? Test out stevia! Make a nice-sized fruit bowl and mix either sugar-free probiotic yogurt or full-fat coconut milk with a packet or two of stevia. Plop on your fake whipped cream (the yogurt or coconut milk) and maybe toast a few coconut shavings. Want to really do it right? Shaved almonds will add protein and more healthy fats.

Dairy: Probiotic sugar-free yogurt can support the pancreas and assure that all aspects of your digestion keep percolating along. If you struggle with pancreatic issues—kind of a thing for overstressed

Thinkers—refrain from full-fat dairy products, margarine, butter, ghee, and mayonnaise. Low- or nonfat dairy should be absolutely fine (if you are okay with dairy); just keep your milk natural and organic.

There are mixed reviews about the health effects of cow dairy on the digestive system. In infants, it's quite possible that the molecules of cow dairy are absorbed in the permeable intestinal tract and are seen as foreign proteins—hence, enemies. Cow dairy could set up your pancreas for problems, such as type 1 diabetes. That's the childhood type. Type 2 is usually adult onset diabetes and has been linked to the overprocessed, bad-fat Western diet. All of this is to say, be super careful about what type of dairy is good for your body and what isn't. (Almond, coconut, hemp, oat, or rice milk are good substitutes for cow dairy.)

Liquids: Dehydration is the Thinker's downfall. So hydrate! Drink at least eight glasses of water a day and abstain from alcohol when possible. Thinkers are prone to desiring dehydrating beverages (think caffeinated and carbonated). Why is this? The bubblies give you a pick-me-up, but it's easy to get hooked on this artificial mood enhancer. In fact, we know lots of Thinkers who drink can after can of soda pop rather than spend the time necessary to figure out the root of the compulsion (which usually is dislike of a job, imbalance in life structure, or overwork). So make smarter choices. Put down the sodas and drink regular water. If you can't avoid the sodas, then drink the bubbly water, but know you aren't getting as hydrated as you might want, so drink regular water too. For any type of water, get fancy by adding lemon or lime for the extra enzyme boost.

Supplements and Spices: Remember Popeye the Sailor Man? (If you don't, you can still find him on YouTube.) He wasn't exactly a Thinker, but his superpowers were turned on under the same conditions: gobbling iron. Consider getting bloodwork to check if you should supplement with iron for power and B vitamins to keep you going. Garlic shows up on many pancreas-healthy diets for its detoxification abilities. Calendula has anti-inflammatory properties, and licorice root supports the pancreas. Goldenseal, horsetail, oregano, dandelion, olive leaves, and even the blue flower gentian, all have healing properties that make them good Thinker choices.

Select other supplements and spices as needed. Liquid minerals, for instance, especially when ionized with sea salt, can aid all the digestive organs. Milk thistle supports the liver and increases inositol, which boosts the effectiveness of B vitamins. Magnesium can lower anxiety, as can choline and lecithin. You can also create a detoxification drink of olive oil, cayenne pepper, lemon juice, parsley, ginger, and pectin. Drink it three times a day for a few days, for up to a week. Drink it sparingly and on an empty stomach—if you can tolerate it—to cleanse your digestive tract. We suggest drinking this near a trash can the first time, just in case.

The Nopes

You know most of your Nopes already. (Haven't we done a good job of sprinkling those in?) Now we'll anchor you with a more complete list.

- The whites. *No whites!* Remember these include all whites: flour, potatoes, white rice, and sugar. And no fake sugars! We're talking aspartame, sucralose, and saccharin.

- Fried foods and fatty fats. Not good for the pancreas. There, we've said it three times.

- Alcohol. Best avoided. It's hard on your entire digestive system to process out all those toxins.

- Sodas. Those bubblies, especially if there is caffeine or sugar in them, will help you pretend away the negatives. That's not a real fix, though. (Maybe try therapy? Or hang around happy people? Okay, worst case, drink carbonated water.)

- Processed foods. Who said processed food is food? It isn't. It's chemicals and preservatives that do you no good. Goodbye to food dyes, artificial flavors, and the rest.

- Caffeine—unless you use it judiciously. A lot of Thinkers make their caffeine do their emotional work for them. If you really hate what you're doing, don't force yourself forward with the caffeine. Think of a better plan and execute it. New job? Better work environment? Happier home? Go for it.

REAL-LIFE EATING TIPS

How are you going to figure out how to fix all these great foods for yourself? Or when, if in need of a break, you should eat out? It's time to find out.

Food Prep

Details, details, details. They are your forte. So, let's get at them.

Overall, make a plan. In fact, create a contract with yourself and keep it, sort of like this:

- Make your weekly breakfast and dinner plans every Saturday. Then shop for the week. (See the next section on that matter.)

- Prep on Sundays. Cut and chop, cook and sauté, bag and freeze. Label. Establish your eating schedule, especially what you'll do for lunch each day. (Overworker that you are, it's tempting for you to skip lunch. Best if you don't.)

- Package your snacks. Small glass containers or some eco-friendly wrap will hold the snacks you put together. Remember to mix a vegetable, protein, and fat when possible.

- Select your cheat food. You're human. Figure out what you'll indulge in when you're feeling down. Dark chocolate? Buy that bar on Saturday and save it. A frozen fruit bar? Same. Plan on *one* cheat food a week (okay, we're pretty strict) and you'll be fine.

Grocery Shopping

Grocery shopping is fun for you—as long as you go to a store that has everything or you plan on shopping at two stores. Before you go shopping, make your list according to the already provided categories: proteins, fats, carbs, vegetables and fruit, dairy, liquids, supplements, and spices. Then add in your etceteras, like snacks and that (single) cheat food.

Thinkers also have this unusual habit: they buy better food if they're better dressed. Don't shop in your hang-out sweats. The more businesslike your attire, the more aligned your choices will be.

Dining Out

To enjoy dining out, you've got to first deal with your analytic (let's be honest—anal) nature. Select a restaurant that takes reservations and presents a clear, detailed menu. Going to restaurants that change their menus whenever they feel like it can be stressful. You like punctuality, including attentive waitstaff, so keep that in mind. Consider inviting companions who can read a clock and don't want to linger longer than you do.

BONUS MATERIAL—BEYOND FOOD

You can select the correct foods and follow protocol, but also support your health with activities that suit your chakra type.

Exercise and Movement

You can basically perform any exercise as long as you plan ahead. We recommend you establish a routine that rotates aerobic and anaerobic exercises. Want to go aerobic? Think sustained activity, like biking, fast walking, or swimming. How about Pilates or yoga for anaerobic? Or create a home gym and go for it in your house or apartment. It's sure to fit your schedule that way.

Mindfulness and Spiritual Practices

Who would have imagined that you might actually be interested in something like intuitive development? You are a mental empath. You also love learning. Your mind gets so chatty that by combining a path of intuitive development and training you'll become quite . . . Zen. You can also apply your mental empathy to deciding what to eat using the following technique.

EXERCISE: MENTAL EMPATHY AND FOOD CHOICES
Take a few deep breaths and connect with your inner sage. Then do the following:

1. Focus on your food desire. Imagine that you are holding it in your hand or looking at it.
2. Go with your gut. Deep inside your solar plexus, you'll sense whether you should eat it or not. Basically, your bodily energy will rise upward and your mind will quiet if it's a yes. Your physical stamina will fall downward and your mind will chit-chat if it's a no.
3. Follow this guidance.

Sleep and Relaxation
It's all about routine and knowing what to do when you break it. Take these actions:

1. Establish a set rising time, bedtime, and nighttime routine. Plan everything, down to which days you go to the gym or take a walk.
2. Keep the same set times every week or workday. You thrive on ritual.
3. Set a notepad next to the bed for the thoughts that wake you in the middle of the night. Jot down those intrusive ideas, and you'll fall asleep again. Use a lamp and not your phone for light, however, as you may be tempted to check your emails.
4. Sleep with the same pillow or stuffed object most of the time.

(We're trying to avoid calling it a teddy bear.) Even though you're a Thinker, you need some cozy comfort. Plus, we're setting you up for the next recommendation.

5. When your routine is disturbed because you're traveling—or you are simply way stressed out—take your pillow on the trip. The only downside is that you might not have enough room in your carry-on for the traveling pillow. Then again, you're a very organized packer. Packing cubes will change your life.

Stress-busting and Prevention

One of the quickest ways for you to stop fretting is to go yellow. Think yellow. Picture yellow. Wear yellow. Heck, eat a banana! They're yellow and have a lot of minerals. Besides that, you need a bucket of tools for mind control to stop the craziness in your overactive head. We recommend you check out Neuro-Linguistic Programming (NLP). It approaches experiences as neither good nor bad, thus getting you out of negativity and judgmentalism. The practice then helps you logically decide how to approach a situation and yourself. Besides that, distract yourself. Overwhelmed during a meeting? Walk to the coffee room or around the block. Feeling down on yourself? Go get on the swings at a park.

Self-Care Rituals and Needs

As a Thinker, you'll want to approach self-care in two opposite ways. Because you're analytical, you need a ritual that is logical and detailed. You also need to feel sky high and carefree.

Totally recommended? A tidying program. The cleaner your space, the cleaner your thoughts. As soon as possible, compose a decluttering program. Set a schedule, perhaps basing it on hours per week and the order of rooms to go through. Then go at it. You can also try out an already existing decluttering program. We're huge fans of Marie Kondo; she even provides a checklist.

Then, think outside of the box. *Way* outside. You have to wander and wonder. Suggestions? Sit down every week and perform freestyle writing for fifteen minutes. Don't rein yourself in; just scribble and scratch and embrace the messy self who emerges. Or, select an off-style article of clothing to wear. In general, you like crisp, clean, and tailored clothing. So at least once a week, wear a smock, multicolored golf pants, or unmatched socks; let the artist in you emerge. You'll better appreciate the more creative folks in your life and maybe even (sort of) become one.

SELF-ASSESSMENT QUESTIONS

In order to build your chakra map in part III, you'll want to pick and choose from the concepts and tips provided in this chapter. Spend some time focusing on these questions, and take notes if you can.

1. What's one personal trait that you wish to fully embrace and build on?
2. What's a weakness that you now know to be watchful for?
3. Which foods from the recommended list are your favorites and should be included in your plan?
4. Which foods from the Nopes list do you need to take out of your current diet?
5. What are some possible substitutions for the Nope foods that you could eat instead?
6. What do you fear could be the trip-up point, or downfall, of your new plan? Is there a professional or someone you know who could help you with that?
7. Take stock of your current pantry and food items. Are there any items you should toss out so as not to be tempted?
8. What recommended supplements do you already use, or want to start using, to support your health?
9. Which of the quick tips and real-life tips do you want to use?

10. What grocery shopping and dining habits can you change to help you follow your new plan?

And a few extra questions:

1. What are two forms of exercise mentioned for your type that appeal to you?
2. What one mindfulness or relaxation technique can you implement when stressed?
3. How about sleep? Is there a way you can improve it? Can you plan better to dedicate more time for nodding off?
4. Select a self-care ritual you know you'll do.
5. Is there another chakra that you would like to strengthen within yourself? If so, what foods or activities can you implement from that specific type to help bolster that chakra within you?

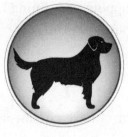

7

RELATER

Purpose: To Relate
Love. For you, that's what it's all about. You're dialed in to the relationships among all people and beings. Ultimately, you're constantly assessing your world for the presence or absence of love.

Chakra Location: Heart
Of course you're centered in the heart. Actually, you're anchored in your heart chakra, which is in the center of the chest. Also in the area of this chakra are the pericardium, breasts, and lungs, as well as the cardiac plexus—a group of nerves connected to the fight-flight-freeze-fawn reactions—and all things that go lub-dub.

Color: Green
Don't you love the fresh burst of green in spring? Green is considered a color reflective of love and healing. Like love itself, green promises new beginnings.

Chakra Affirmation:
I am lovable and have healthy relationships.

RELATER PERSONALITY TRAITS

Delighting in relationships, you are the love child of the chakra universe. Love fuels your being. You also tend to pick your foodstuffs in the same freestyle way. Left untended, you'll eat what you love and avoid what you don't. Sometimes that works and sometimes it doesn't. We'll get that sorted out. Let's take a look.

> **WORDS TO DESCRIBE YOUR RELATER SELF:**
> Lover. Relationship focused. Heart centered.
> Connector. Affectionate. Helper. Caring. Healer.

Your main intuitive gift is relational empathy. What a lovely intuitive gift: to be able to sense the energy of love. There is no higher gift.

Through relationship empathy, you can psychically sense the nature of another's relationship with self, others, and the Spirit. You can even stretch in another direction: toward healing. Think back. How many times have you simply "known" about other people's issues, illnesses, and needs and what might restore them to wholeness?

We want to teach you how to employ your intuitive gift to help others heal, and how to create inner wholeness by finding the foods that will love you. We'll accomplish that through the exercise called "Relational Empathy and Food Choices" found later in this chapter.

Your major motivator is to create love. You consider yourself successful if your interactions leave everyone in a higher state of love. That sad friend of yours? You offer them more than compassion; you provide them the needed experience of feeling loved.

Your hidden fear is of intimacy. And yet it's what you long for above all else. Wrapped up in this fear is the worry that you aren't lovable. Because of this fear, you may find yourself in codependent relationships or engaging in codependent activities. Work on receiving love and trusting yourself to take care of your own heart.

Your greatest strength is your healing ability. The word "healing" means "to make whole." Love shows us the wholeness that endures beneath the illusion of brokenness. You are an amplifier of that love through your ability to collaborate and partner with others. Build on that strength and these qualities:

- Unifying. Love is the binding force of the universe. The people, animals, and even plants in your sphere know you as a great connector.

- Sharing. What wouldn't you give to—or do for—someone you love? When aligned with your integrity, you're an unconditional soul.

- Intimate. Dissected, the word intimacy means "into you, into me." You desire nothing but oneness with those you care about.

- Unconditional lover. You know that love can change the world, or even the mood of a single coffee barista.

- Heroic. You can see (and act) beyond the danger and fear inherent in a situation. If another can be healed or saved, you will heroically save them.

Your greatest weakness is that you want to heal everyone. We commend your ability to take care of others. However, over-caretaking, also called codependency, can be your downfall. Codependency can be defined as doing for others what they should do for themselves. But it also involves doing for others what isn't good for *you*.

Apply this tendency to food. Cyndi has a great story to make the point.

Every summer, she and her family went to visit her Great-Uncle Andrew and Great-Aunt Hannah in Fargo, North Dakota. Hannah would make strawberry shortcake: the worst version ever. The biscuits, dry. The strawberries, freezer-burned: pale and mushy. Cyndi hated that shortcake. But her mom insisted she eat it all, lest she hurt Hannah's feelings. Then, as if that weren't bad enough, she was forced to eat seconds to protect Hannah yet again.

These are the types of situations Relaters often find themselves in. They can too easily cook, eat, select menu items, and even grocery shop so as to not hurt others. Does your partner feel lonely if you no longer share their favorite dessert or after-dinner drink? Is your mom upset because she can't fix you your favorite childhood dinner anymore? You see what we mean.

Want to know a few more of your weaknesses? Here you go:

- Grandiosity: Just because you know what someone might require for healing doesn't mean you're the expert.

- Love addiction. Love feels good—unless it's not really love. If a relationship makes you feel bad, it's not good.

- Giving-receiving imbalances. It feels so good to give that you can forget to receive. You might even be downright scared to receive, because when you're receiving, you lose control.

- Taking other people's issues personally. What if someone thinks it's your fault that you can't fix them? Fill in the holes in their heart? You aren't responsible for another's responsibilities, or even their feelings.

Achieving a harmonious weight. Is your weight out of whack? If so, the root cause is most likely an imbalance in love. Give love away with nothing coming back, and you'll reach for food to fill up. Only taking, and not giving? You may be underweight *or* overeat because you don't believe you deserve both parts of the give-take cycle. Dangerous or abusive relationships nearly always cause erratic weight. Every time someone treats you badly, you'll either reach for food or starve yourself toward a perceived idea of perfection or invisibility. You need to love yourself before you engage in a loving relationship.

Codependency, fueled by fear of loss, can also lead to weight imbalances. If you're over-focused on others, you're under-focused on your own nourishment. See a therapist if your fear of not being enough, or of being abandoned, compels poor decisions.

Your chakra endocrine gland is your heart: you make all ***your food choices with this gland in mind.*** Until recently, Westerners failed to recognize what Eastern mystics have always known: the heart is a major endocrine gland. In fact, it might even be *the* major endocrine gland, making hormones like oxytocin, the bonding hormone. Its rhythm and protocol likely determine the health and well-being of all other hormone-producing glands too, including the brain.

The heart's energetic field is the major generator of electromagnetism. In fact, it emanates an electromagnetic field 50,000 times greater than does the brain. That means that as a Relater, you can literally sense what others are feeling and needing, even from a distance. So it's all the more important to keep your heart stable.

There is more to the heart than physical energy. Research from organizations including HeartMath Inc. in California shows that the healthy heart isn't only dependent on good nutrition and exercise. To be in optimum condition, it must also be filled with intangibles like love, faith, and hope. The heart is hurt by situations that aren't based on these spiritual qualities. In fact, you have a higher risk of developing cardiovascular issues if you've lived through abuse or violence of any sort.

We've found that individuals with hurting hearts often make poor food choices. The good news is that love has the power to heal. If you decide that self-love wins over hurt and pain, you can shift your diet to wield great results.

FOOD AND SUPPLEMENT PROGRAM
FOR THE THINKER

Now it's time to dive into some food-related tips specifically for you. Included is a list of the fourth-chakra body parts and the metaphysical explanation of them as well. This way, if you struggle with a particular food, you can work on the related emotional issue.

Quick Tips and Tricks for the Thinker

Let's dig into the specific ways to love up your heart.

1. Assess for food allergies and sensitivities. If you need to, employ a physician, cardiologist, allergist, nutritionist, or naturopath.
2. Don't make choices out of love-euphoria or love-misery. When you're in bliss, it's easy to toss common sense out and snack with your lover on pastries and desserts. Feeling miserable?

CASE STUDY: MAURICE

Maurice was willing to eat a heart-healthy diet. Sort of. What he wasn't eager to do was give up his wine and "smokes." Or the fried foods and comforting desserts. He especially loved biscuits and ice cream. Though not at the same time.

When asked about his sense of life purpose, he smiled and said, "Making sure the woman I love is happy, that everyone in my family is taken care of." Then his smile faded, and he looked away. The truth was, Maurice was constantly trying to make his depressed wife happy, but it never seemed to work. He felt responsible for her emotional state and was drowning his own feelings of loneliness in fatty foods and alcohol.

Maurice understood that a lot of his habits were unhealthy, but he was scared of giving them up. "Food is the only thing that brings me happiness. How will I have anything to look forward to if I give up the food I love?" he asked. So we worked with him on his feelings before altering his behaviors. It was time to deal with the emotions locked inside his heart chakra.

It didn't take long to figure out that Maurice was a heart-based people pleaser. As his parents' firstborn, he was afflicted with a deep and undeserved guilt about keeping them together. They argued all the time, he explained. In fact, they never let up. They had lost a child when Maurice was young, and he assumed the role of being his mom's best friend and providing comfort. Maurice's breakthrough moment was when he realized he constantly took care of others (like his mom) to try to get his own needs met. It never worked, so he indulged in pleasures like food, drink, and smoking because he felt like *he* "deserved" the joy he gave away to others.

After achieving this awareness, Maurice became willing to deal with his smoking. He employed a hypnotist—and dissolved into a puddle of emotions. For days. He became aware of how he reached for friendly foods when he craved intimacy and connection. We taught him ways to connect to himself; he particularly enjoyed journaling and a men's group he joined that focused on sharing and connection. After that, he found it much easier to start abstaining from his other cravings and substituting heart-healthy foods. Eventually, he reduced his wine and ice cream consumption to a reasonable amount that felt comfortable without being overindulgent.

He then began to look more closely at his relationship and suggested to his wife that they see a marriage therapist. She agreed, and they started working diligently on their issues. He began learning to be responsible for his own needs and emotions, and to let his wife be responsible for hers. This led her to blossom as well, especially after she was diagnosed with clinical depression and was able to find the right treatment. It came as a relief when he realized it truly wasn't his job to maintain her happiness. Together, they focused on eating healthy and connecting through grocery shopping and prepping food together. When either wanted to eat cheat foods, they would go for a long walk, holding hands, and talk instead.

Eventually Maurice felt so strong in his partnership and in his healthy eating habits that he signed up for a hands-on healing class. Yes, underneath his challenging patterns were an emerging heart and a healer.

Heartbroken or in grief? Put down the ice cream and alcohol. Process your feelings. Follow your plan.

3. Adopt the Mediterranean diet. Consume lots of veggies, fruits, whole grains, and healthy fats. Moderate your intake of fish, poultry, beans, and eggs, as well as dairy. And limit your consumption of red meat. Your best diet is plant-based, or as plant-based as can be.

4. Eat meat as a side dish rather than the main meal.

5. Know your portions. One stalk of asparagus isn't a full serving of veggies, and one huge ice cream cone is more than one serving of dairy.

6. Food combine—your way. Combine a healthy grain or starch with a protein and a fat every time you eat. Here are a couple of extra ideas to follow:

   • Combine fibrous foods (such as oats, beans, veggies) with plant sterols (like beans, legumes, nuts, soy, and seeds).

   • Mix olive oil and tomato sauce. It will increase your absorption of lycopene, which we cover under "Vegetables and Fruits."

   • Stir together seafood and strawberries—or any heme iron sourced food (animal, poultry, seafood) with a non–heme iron (plant-based)-sourced food. By putting them together, you get better absorption of both.

- Blend rice and beans.

7. Then there is the "don't combine" category. Certain food groupings cancel out heart benefits. Try to avoid these combos:
    - B-vitamin foods and animal foods. (So don't eat a steak or sausage with your breakfast cereal.)
    - B-vitamin foods and coffee or alcohol. (No toast and beer or café au lait.)
    - Folic acid and wine. (No asparagus and red wine.)

8. Start with self-love. If you give yourself away, do you know what you'll do? Eat and drink to fill up the hole. If you're whole, there aren't any holes.

9. Drink lots of water.

10. About that chocolate. We might confuse you a little in this chapter. At some points, we say, "Watch for chocolate." Other times, we'll tell you it's a fantastic extra treat. What we mean is that moderation is key. Dark chocolate is your friend if nibbled twice a week.

11. The heart chakra bodily organs and parts have metaphysical meanings. Sometimes you reach for food when you're afflicted with emotional issues. Here are some connections to get familiar with—and to get healing for, if needed.
    - Heart: Issues about love will cause you to reach for sugar, wine, soft and soothing carbs, and overly fatty foods. You'll specifically crave wine or chocolate if you don't have the romance you desire.
    - Breasts: These hold issues about maternal love—or the lack thereof. In later life, breasts can hold issues about partnership/romantic love. Cravings for ice cream, candy, and soft carbs such as cookies, pies, and cakes will surface.
    - Lungs: The lungs reflect your relationship with the Spirit,

and also hold unresolved grief. Here comes the desire for tobacco, fruit juices, and sugary products.

- Pericardium: The heart protector. When you're not feeling safe or lovable, you'll go for foods that congest and produce mucus, like dairy or gluten. These foods can also keep you from expressing your emotions, which might be trapped in the heart.

FOOD CATEGORIES

Now, to cover the choices you can make within the various food categories.

Proteins: We have lots of heart-healthy protein advice—just don't take it with many grains of salt, as that's not your best spice. If you're a meat eater, eat small amounts of extra-lean ground beef or ground turkey breast. Trim those fatty cuts—or don't buy them. To keep your fleshy protein lean, bake your chicken and fish without skin, and grill your steaks.

Speaking of fish, recommended are fatty fish like salmon, mackerel, sardines, and tuna. The omega-3s in fatty fish are heart healthy in every way. Seafood in general is pretty heart healthy: shrimp, crab, scampi, mussels, and crayfish. Eat up. Just don't fry them. Pair them with healthy greens and oils, and your heart—and stomach—will thank you. See the Shrimp Salad recipe in this chapter.

Want to go vegan or reduce your consumption of fleshy proteins? That's a great idea for the Relater. Eat moderate amounts of beans and legumes; we'll cover these more in the carb section. For nuts, think walnuts. Adding a few servings to your diet protects against heart disease and adds fiber. Almonds are loaded with needed vitamins and minerals, the good monounsaturated fats, and fiber, and can boost your healthy cholesterol and reduce the bad kind. Your heart also gets happy with chia, flax, and hemp seeds. Sprinkle shaved nuts or seeds over the least desirable part of a meal to make it more enjoyable.

Plant protein substitutes can make your heart happy. Buckwheat, quinoa, hemp hearts, and soy-based foods like tempeh and tofu can be good options.

SHRIMP SALAD

Add some olive oil to a hot pan and toss in a serving's worth of peeled shrimp to sear. Lay the cooked shrimp over a bed of fresh spinach. Dice some strawberries and crush a few walnuts. Sprinkle both over top. Dust with goat feta. Drizzle generously with olive oil and lemon. You can add a dash or two of balsamic vinegar if you want an extra punch.

Fats: Two words: Olive oil. That's the oil most used in the Mediterranean countries, and the best for your health. Dip your veggies in it, and drizzle salads with it.

In general, you want to reach for these three main types of fats: omega-3 fatty acids, monounsaturated fats, and polyunsaturated fats. Omega-3s are found in oily fish like tuna, salmon, and the list of those covered in the proteins section. You can also go for the nuts and seeds mentioned there. Don't cook with these oils, however. For cooking, choose oils with monounsaturated fats, like canola and peanut oil. You can also use avocado oil. It has a high smoke point, so it's great for cooking.

What about the polyunsaturated fats? These can lower LDL cholesterol. Go for vegetable oils to meet this need, including safflower, sunflower, sesame, soybean, and corn.

Here is what you want to abstain from, or seriously limit: saturated fats, such as those in meats and dairy—except! Read the dairy section. Full-fat dairy can be beneficial. Just limit yourself. Trans fats, like partially and fully hydrogenated oils, will clog your system. (Goodbye processed foods.) Dump the coconut or palm oil, margarine, lard, overuse of butter, and bacon fat.

Carbohydrates: Think whole and you'll have a "whole," or healed, heart. If you can eat gluten, start with getting three servings of whole grains every day. These can help keep the heart doctor away. Types include whole wheat or rye bread, high-fiber cereals, barley and buckwheat, whole-grain pastas, and oatmeal. Don't do gluten? Go for brown rice or non-gluten bread loaded with seeds and nuts. (Sorry, white biscuits and gravy are on the "no" list. Avoid white rice too.)

Then on to beans. They contain resistant starch, which aids digestion and feeds the good bacteria in your gut. This type of starch can improve heart health. Legumes are good too. In fact, try chili. Throw in a protein, two or three cans of beans, and then borrow from our next category and add tomatoes, carrots, and corn. Honestly, you don't even need to be a meat eater. Beans have protein. Pair that bowl of chili with avocado on whole-grain toast drizzled in olive oil, and your heart will be smiling before you take the first bite.

Vegetables and Fruits: Eat lots of both. Leafy green vegetables like kale, collard greens, chard, and spinach lower your risk of heart disease. They also give you a super-shot of vitamin K, which boosts arterial health and proper blood clotting. In addition, leafy greens feature dietary nitrates, which boost your heart health. The cruciferous vegetables are also terrific; load up on broccoli, cauliflower, brussels sprouts, bok choy, and cabbage.

Eat avocados for the win. They give you great fats and are versatile. Don't skip the tomatoes. They're an antioxidant, and the lycopene in them is associated with a reduced risk of heart disease and stroke. If you go fruit, eat berries: strawberries, blueberries, blackberries, raspberries. All are good for your heart, and you can add in oranges, cantaloupe, and papaya. Actually, just think fruit, period. A fun little trick? Pick fruits that are heart-shaped. Most berries are!

Want to really go Mediterranean? Start your day with a breakfast smorgasbord of veggies and fruits. Select from purple grapes, sliced tomatoes and cucumbers, feta cheese, hummus, and a whole-grain or gluten-free pita bread. Eat, then pack the rest for a later snack. Or go Nordic and eat a breakfast of whole-grain seeded bread with salmon, cheese, and fresh veggies and fruits.

Dairy: Sometimes milk gets a bad name. (Inflammatory, creates allergens, produces mucus.) For a Relater? Guess what? Milk products are linked with a reduced risk of cardiovascular diseases, including hypertension, stroke, and coronary artery disease. Test first to be sure you're not lactose or casein intolerant. Hint: if you have to use the bathroom every time you consume cow dairy, you're likely intolerant.

Best choices? The higher-fat ones, such as cheese. You can include yogurt; just don't pick the sugary types. Also try feta and goat cheese.

Liquids: The heart loves water. After all, an adult has 100,000 miles of blood vessels in their body—all powered by water. That means your cardiovascular systems needs a lot of it. Aim for eight to ten glasses a day.

You can also go for low-fat milk or soy milk, and if you have high cholesterol, consider sterol-fortified fruit juices (without sugar, and only four ounces at a time). Then give the go-ahead to tea, especially green tea. It seems to reduce the risk of strokes and heart attacks and can lower total and LDL cholesterol. We don't mean sweet tea.

Lots of people believe coffee is heart-healthy. Make your own decision, but if you drink it, go for black coffee and avoid the lattes. A little red wine is fine once in a while, but soda and cola? Your physical heart says yuck.

Supplements and Spices: The good news is that the Relater's heart adores supplements and spices. Using either can help reduce cravings for the Nopes and keep your heart muscle beating strong.

Often recommended for heart health are omega-3 supplements, such as fish and cod liver oil capsules. You can also check out krill and algal oil supplements. You also want to be conscious of your omega-3 and omega-6 ratios. The ratio should be 1:4, respectively. Flax seeds provide omega-6. Want a powerhouse supplement for the heart? Select coenzyme Q10, an enzyme for your mitochondria, your inner cellular energy factories. As well, astaxanthin has super anti-inflammatory effects and assists with maintaining normal cholesterol levels.

We can't say enough about magnesium for heart health. Watch it, though, if you have kidney disease, and work with a professional to see what type you need. You can also use a magnesium gel or lotion to bring magnesium straight into your bloodstream through the skin.

A lot of Relaters like L-carnitine too. It's an amino acid. Guess what it does? It brings fats into your mitochondria and will help oxygenate you too.

A word of caution: you might want to watch your choline, meaning don't get excessive amounts of it. It's ingested through meat, eggs, and milk, so limit those foods, and maybe don't supplement. Choline may raise the levels of a bacteria-producing compound that could form clots.

Of course, you've lots of organs in your heart chakra. For your breasts, check out vitamin D, probiotics, sulforaphane (it's in broccoli, so that makes it easier), and N-acetylcysteine, a major antioxidant. Your lungs also love vitamin D, as well as the full array of the "normal" vitamins, like B, C, and E.

Heart-happy spices include cayenne pepper, garlic, hawthorn, and turmeric. The lungs like garlic, hawthorn, and shiitake mushrooms. The latter are superb for reducing the incidence of common lung complaints. But your pantry can include a lot of other spices and herbs. A short list includes basil, bay leaves, black pepper, caraway

seeds, chili powder, ginger, cinnamon, cloves, nutmeg, oregano, paprika, and parsley.

The Nopes

Overall, inflammatory foods aren't good for any of the heart chakra
organs. Here are a few specifics:

- The whites. White rice, white breads, white sugars. You get the picture.

- Sugars. Whites and fakes. Avoid them.

- Tobacco. Metaphysically, Relaters reach for tobacco when feeling
  lonely. Remember: the lungs hold grief, and they also forge a bond
  with the Spirit. If we are lonely or in need of a friend, we might reach
  for cigarettes or chewing tobacco. See our self-care section later for
  alternative ideas.

- Wine. A lot of female Relaters love wine. Energetically, wine is a substitute for romance and connection. Missing those in your life? Out
  comes the wine glass—or an entire bottle. Don't let yourself get too
  lonely; get a real friend (dogs count) instead. Men, watch your beer
  intake when you're feeling lonely.

- Chocolate. Another fix for romance! Don't keep any in the house.
  Only eat chocolate one piece or bar at a time, and do it outside the
  house. *But* limited amounts of dark chocolate help the heart.

- Fried and overly fatty foods and fatty fats. Say goodbye to marbled
  meat cuts, organ meats, chicken tenders, and processed lunch meats.

- Processed foods. These aren't food. They will gum up your blood vessels and your thinking.

- Caffeine, if overused. Sometimes too much caffeine can throw off your
  heart rhythm and, for some people, their blood pressure. Listen to
  your body.

- Too much salt. We know it helps food taste better. Just watch your
  intake.

REAL-LIFE EATING TIPS

It's not enough to know what to eat (and not). If you're going to eat, you have to buy and make the right foods. Want to eat out? We have a few tips for you in this section.

Food Prep

Food preparation isn't exactly your thing, unless you have help or company. If you do it alone, you'll lose energy. Do you have someone who will prep with you once or twice a week? Maybe chat with you while you're fixing dinner? Short of a real-life person, talk with your pet. If you have food anywhere in the kitchen, a dog will happily stare at you—and follow your every movement. Utilize technology for help and company. Download a prep session with a super cool chef or find an entertaining cook who showcases all the fun knife tricks and food shortcuts.

Then, for the actual cooking process, don't fry. Bake, steam, or grill. Your heart will thank you.

Grocery Shopping

Food, food everywhere—and no one to help you make a selection. That's going to stump you, and you'll buy what you shouldn't, like fatty meat, cinnamon buns, and wine.

You are a people person. A lover of love. How about creating your list with a friend, partner, or child? Perhaps you have a friend who likes to cook. Align your meal plans and shopping lists even if you're not dining together. Maybe you could even convince someone to let you text them for advice while you're shopping. If you get healthy input, you'll make healthier choices.

Dining Out

Warning! Dining out is fun, isn't it? You have to watch for two dangers, though. If you're with someone you really like, you'll be apt to go mindless during the eating activity. You'll enjoy the talking instead of paying attention to your body. Think through what you're going to order and order only that item. Pass on dessert. Otherwise, you'll overeat.

What's the other red flag? Relaters can also overeat when eating alone. Lonely opportunities like solo road or business trips can bring on the snacking, drinking, and indulging. If you're out to eat by your-self, bring a book or an activity that will occupy you.

BONUS MATERIAL—BEYOND FOOD

It's not all about the food. Other activities can lead you skipping down the path of health.

Exercise and Movement

In general, do anything that will make your heart beat faster. Pump up your heart rate for thirty minutes once a day. There are lots of ways to do that: bicycle, walk, hike (that means make sure your walk includes a few hills), swim, jog—anything you love. Just get that heart going. You'll really love exercising if you have a partner or friend along. How-ever, just hanging out with a friend (which you love to do) isn't exercise. So plan movement get-togethers like walking through the park or mall, going to the gym or a studio class, or taking an outdoor bike ride, a row on the lake, or a hike.

Mindfulness and Spiritual Practices

We have a simple exercise we'd like you to conduct every day. It's called receiving love.

We know others have hurt you. You have reason to block your heart, but a spiritually and emotionally blocked heart leads to phys-ical blocks—and those pesky food cravings. So picture love in the symbol of the cross (we're not talking religion here).

Imagine the vertical piece of the cross as your connection to the Spirit and unconditional love. People, and all other living beings, bond with you through the horizontal piece. You live at the intersection between perfect and imperfect love.

Each evening hold the image of the cross in your mind's eye and give permission for all the love that has been sent your way during the day to come into your heart. Do so while focusing on this statement:

When I allow in love from imperfect sources, it is accompanied by love from the perfect source.

Whatever is missing in the love from imperfect others will be filled in by that of the Spirit. Of course, you have boundaries. You aren't putting up with abuse or severe negativity (see the lesson on caretaking). But you deserve to absorb love and fill your own heart every night. If you do this regularly, you'll notice a reduction in cravings for unhealthy foods.

The other recommendation? Apply your relational empathy to help you make great food choices! We'll show you how.

Exercise: Relational Empathy and Food Choices

You want to stop *only* selecting foods that you love and choose those that will love you. We'll show you how to use your relational empathy to do this.

1. When you're ready to choose something to eat, sit down for a second and take a few deep breaths. Connect with your inner sage or the Spirit.
2. Think of one of your food ideas. Now imagine that you've already eaten it. Does your system feel satisfied, gratified, and more energized? Or does it seem empty, desirous, and less energized? Go through all the foods and eat only those that provide the first set of results.

Sleep and Relaxation

Here's the thing about a Relater. Whether sleeping or relaxing, they like companionship. Always. But you may not always have a bed friend.

All is well if you have a great sleep or snuggle mate. Except when you're grumpy or they're grumpy, either of you are sick, you're fighting, someone is traveling—you get the idea. Then again, you might be single. Try pillows. If you don't have a partner or a pet, cuddle up with a body pillow.

Watching television? Use a sleep sack. On your days off, have an array of comfy clothes. Flannel is good, as are well-worn sweats.

Stress-busting and Prevention

We have two main stress-busting recommendations. One is external, and the other is internal.

The first is to spend time with a friend. You don't even need the talking kind. Rather, pick a friend who can just hang out with you. Garden, take a walk, go to the zoo, watch the movies. Let go of your problems and everyone else's too.

The second involves breathing. The lungs are found in the fourth chakra. In Eastern medicine, they manage our relationship with the Spirit and hold and process grief. Breathing deeply will provide connection, which gives you a high, and releases emotions. Every so often, breathe in for four counts and hold for four. Then release for seven counts. You can do this two minutes at a time.

Self-Care Rituals and Needs

You're so often taking care of others that your best practices must include taking care of yourself. So, grab a piece of paper. Put the word "Indulgences" on it. The rule is that none of these treats can involve food. Want a list of Relater-loving luxuries? Here we go:

- Massages. Just receive.

- Receive energy healings. Book a session with a great healer. We recommend checking out Healing Touch Program providers, Reiki, faith-based healing, or energy healing.

- Therapy. You spend so much time taking care of others, which includes listening to them. You deserve to have someone listen to you.

- Volunteer for non-people. You'll feel refreshed by spending time volunteering with those beings that only give back—animals.

SELF-ASSESSMENT QUESTIONS

In order to build your chakra map in part III, you'll want to pick and choose from the concepts and tips provided in this chapter. Spend some time focusing on these questions, and take notes if you can.

1. What's one personal trait that you wish to fully embrace and build on?
2. What's a weakness that you now know to be watchful for?
3. Which foods from the recommended list are your favorites and should be included in your plan?
4. Which foods from the Nopes list do you need to take out of your current diet?
5. What are some possible substitutions for the Nope foods?
6. What do you fear could be the trip-up point, or downfall, of your new plan? Is there a professional or someone you know who could help you with that?
7. Take stock of your current pantry and food items. Are there any items you should toss out so as not to be tempted?
8. What recommended supplements do you already use, or want to start using, to support your health?
9. Which of the quick tips and real-life tips do you want to use?
10. What grocery shopping and dining habits can you change to help you follow your new plan?

And a few extra questions:

1. What are two forms of exercise mentioned for your type that appeal to you?
2. What one mindfulness or relaxation technique can you implement when stressed?

3. How about sleep? Is there a way you can improve it? Can you plan better to dedicate more time to nodding off?
4. Select a self-care ritual you know you'll do.
5. Is there another chakra that you would like to strengthen within yourself? If so, what foods or activities can you implement from that specific type to help bolster that chakra within you?

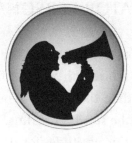

8

COMMUNICATOR

Purpose: To Communicate
You live to communicate, no matter how you do it: learning, teaching, speaking, writing, singing, making music, contemplating. Any form. You also love to learn and teach as a form of communication.

Chakra Location: Thyroid
This small organ in the throat area is especially active for the Communicator, who is incessantly verbalizing, whether internally or externally. It's anchored in the cervical vertebrae, and when it comes to food choices, it can be picky.

Color: Blue
Blue reflects the giving and receiving of information for higher purposes.

Chakra Affirmation:
I am honest and clear in communications with myself and others.

COMMUNICATOR PERSONALITY TRAITS

Ever attuned to the verbal world, you can hear a pin drop while on the phone with a friend, or a bird chirping a mile away. Then again, you might be a lot weirder than that. As in—you're a channeler and can hear information from the spiritual realms. You'll love learning how to use your communication aptitudes for making healthy decisions.

The call to communicate has many facets, as the following discussion of Communicator qualities reveals.

> **WORDS TO DESCRIBE YOUR COMMUNICATOR**
> **SELF:** Talkative. Observant. Loud. Entertaining. Teacher. Outspoken. Opinionated. Curious.

Your main intuitive gift is clairaudience. You have the capacity to "clearly hear," which is what the word "clairaudience" means. This ability gets a lot of press time, even on television, where we meet the gifted who can read minds or talk to the dead. Whether you use these psychic terms in public or not, you are likely a channeler, medium, and telepath.

That doesn't mean you hear voices. A clairaudient might simply read into what another is sharing (or not), pick cool quotes out of books, speak the right words just when needed, receive verbal messages in dreams, or simply have truths pop into their head. Then again, there *is* that tendency to chat with dead people.

Let's not stop here! You have two other intuitive abilities. Clairgustance is the paranormal gift for tasting something without putting it in your mouth. (Ah! What a great diet. Pretend you're eating French fries without eating them.) Clairalience allows you to smell something that's not present. How useful might that be? (Pretend a freshly baked chocolate chip cookie smells like a skunk.) Later in this chapter, we'll provide two exercises designed to help you make peace with and benefit from all three gifts.

Your major motivator is to learn. You love higher truths. You'll read, write, sing, watch, ruminate, speak, or converse your way into and through philosophy, literature, documentaries, and anything else that adds to the body of knowledge you're interested in. Besides learning, you want to share.

Your hidden fear is of boldly expressing yourself. You long to be heard, yet you fear alienating others with your truthful communication. Because of this, you may find yourself holding your tongue or withdrawing when you have something important to say. Work on speaking from the heart. You can't alienate the people who really love and support you.

Your greatest strength is your commitment to truth. You are a truth knower and truth teller. Every sound you hear, word you speak, or phrase you utter is a vote for truth. And you've other talents too:

- Expressiveness. You can't help communicating. Express it all, even when you're emotionally triggered.

- Storytelling. Your voice can paint pictures, whether fiction or nonfiction. Each holds the potential to change the world.

- Enthusiasm. Yeah! You can impress and influence with every engagement.

- Language savvy. The correct words and inflections are at your beck and call. Draw from this potential, whether speaking to yourself or another, to create and motivate change.

- Advice. Whether the messages you deliver come from an invisible guide, a book, or your own mind, you draw on a wellspring of wisdom. You are "listen worthy."

Your greatest weakness is being too impressionable. Just because you can bring forth the voice of authority doesn't mean you're always right. Nor should you be *the* speaker in all situations, or say everything you think. Keep these challenging traits in mind:

- Dishonesty. You could so want to impress someone that you might lie. Oops.

- Honesty. Then again, you probably believe it's your job to say things exactly like they are. (A good rule of thumb? Unless someone asks, don't tell.)

- Compulsive eating. Yup! You can compulsively communicate, so who's to say you won't continually fill your mouth?

- Psychic susceptibility. There are unlimited numbers of invisible beings that might seek to influence you. You can become prey to any of these, and not even know it.

- Fudging. That's what it's called if your "nos" don't always mean "no," and your "yeses" don't always mean "yes." Get clear and be clear, or you'll use food to stuff your truths.

- Anxiety. What are you going to say? Should you talk or not? Be truthful or lie? Share what a spiritual guide offers or not? All that ruminating can lead to anxiety.

Achieving a harmonious weight. Reaching a healthy set point is about living in and expressing the truth. If you hold back, you'll eat to keep everything "stuffed down." If you over-share, perhaps to the point of TMI (too much information), vulnerability, or meanness, you'll abstain from eating as a punishment. Be attuned to the energy of frustration. It can be common in expressive communicators who feel stifled or try to swallow their feelings, words, truths, or opinions to keep peace. Frustration can lead you to stuffing your mouth so you don't talk (or yell) and holding excess weight to protect your true, unexpressed self. Everything in life depends on a balanced cycle: listening and speaking, giving and receiving. And for you, it also depends on honesty, with yourself and others.

Your chakra endocrine gland is your thyroid gland. Make all *your food choices with this gland in mind.* This tiny organ in the throat area is much more powerful than its size would indicate. The hard-working thyroid secretes hormones that control or influence metabolism, weight, growth, mood, energy levels, body temperature, heart rate, and blood pressure. It's busy.

When the thyroid is "off," two main issues can potentially arise. With hypothyroidism, the thyroid doesn't produce enough hormones. You might feel sluggish and not be hungry, yet still gain weight. Or your thyroid can swing toward hyperthyroidism, which means it over-functions. You might gobble up the calories but still lose weight. While a lot of us might like to have the latter problem, it's not good for your body. You'll be wired and tired all the time.

CASE STUDY: ALPHA

Alpha was a professional speaker who assigned herself the name "Alpha" to represent her thirst for success. "I want to reach two million people within ten years," she vowed.

The main problem was that she couldn't stop snacking. Ever. It didn't matter what food was around; it made its way into her mouth. Her body size showed her anxious eating habits.

At some level, Alpha was the consummate Communicator. She even made her living communicating, and loved doing so. In fact, she struggled with turning down speaking engagements, even when they didn't match her expertise. Pretty much, admitted Alpha, she never used the "no" button on her voice box.

Before addressing her diet, we sent Alpha to a physician for

From a subtle point of view, there are energetic factors that can make or break the thyroid. The fifth chakra is the point for channeling higher truths. Messages from the beyond enter through the back side of the throat chakra and are then shared through the front side. This act, called "channeling," is the basis of great works of literature, worldly religions, musical compositions, and great teachings. However, there are health hazards to this channeling activity.

Psychic intrusions can strain the body. Think of it: if you are bringing energy (or beings) into your body that are not your own, you are overloading the thyroid. Eventually, this over-activity can contribute to hyperthyroidism. Your poor little thyroid has to overwork just to keep up with someone else's business! Let's say you shut down the back side of your fifth chakra so you can get some quiet. With half that chakra shut down, your thyroid function might become hypothyroidism. Some Communicators swing between these two extremes. Use the exercise "Getting a Gatekeeper" to acquire some safety and stability.

---

a thyroid test. As expected, she had hypothyroidism. She began working with a naturopath to select the correct supplements. She then stopped eating gluten and dairy and began to curb her eating to focus on lots of veggies, fruits, and lean proteins. To her delight, she discovered that she loved fatty fish, and became quite the chef when composing meal plans around proteins like salmon and tuna. She also reduced her consumption of goitrogens (substances that induce goiter), such as those found in soy and kale, and discovered she was a lot less achy. In fact, she hadn't even known how much pain she felt in her joints and muscles until it went away. Born in Colombia, she began to create recipes based on her culture, which she discovered supported her newfound dietary habits. Black beans. Brown rice. Stir-fries. And a lot of salmon!

Alpha took our advice and restricted her restaurant choices to

FOOD AND SUPPLEMENT PROGRAM FOR THE COMMUNICATOR

Read up on the quick tips for a healthy-eating Communicator.

Quick Tips and Tricks for the Communicator

What keeps a Communicator communicating happily? Here are some foodstuff tips.

1. Follow a diet based on vegetables, fruits, and lean meats. Whole grains are good too—if you keep the Nopes and "mindful moderations" in mind. (You'll learn a lot more about potential dos and don'ts throughout this chapter.)
2. Assess for food allergies and sensitivities. Employ a physician, endocrinologist, allergist, nutritionist, or naturopath if you need to.

---

those serving organic, healthy food, and often preordered so she wouldn't *also* select the food items her husband or a friend might order. And then she started taking yoga classes on Zoom. Equally important, she began cultivating what she came to call her "inner psychic," the quiet voice of spiritual reason that lay within her. Guess what? Her "no" button became available, and she pressed it more often! She found out that the more often she gave a meaningful no, the less often she was prompted to munch. As she became comfortable with the relative quiet—okay, she did play music throughout most of her waking moments—the more spontaneously creative she felt. When last heard from, she was writing a book.

And yes, she has lost a lot of weight since she started her chakra plan, but that wasn't the point of the transformation. Now she's happier and healthier.

3. In general, stay away from foods that cause inflammation or a spike in your blood sugar. That sensitive thyroid also reacts to toxins or chemicals and high amounts of unhealthy fats. That means go organic and hormone-, pesticide-, and antibiotic-free, as well as free-range and wild-caught.

4. Watch out for your oral fixation. Having to constantly move that mouth can lead to smoking, mindless eating and drinking, gum chomping, and even pencil chewing.

5. Know who—or what—you're eating for. You are psychically sensitive, of interest to invisible beings. Are your cravings your own—or do they belong to dead Great-Aunt Hazel, or someone or something else? Clean up your energy using the exercises in this chapter.

6. Turn off the music when eating. Many studies show that people eat less when they eat in silence than when listening to music.

7. Know what to avoid? See if you can say it: goitrogens. These compounds can interfere with the thyroid's function. Especially if you have thyroid troubles, stay away from soy foods and raw vegetables like cabbage, broccoli, and kale; raw fruits and starchy plants; and certain raw nuts and seeds. The exception? You can usually cook with these foods, except for pearl millet. We'll list the Nopes in subsequent categories.

8. Iodine! Iodine is necessary for a fully functional thyroid, and about one-third of the world is iodine deficient. It's found in iodized salt and lots of foods, but you don't want too much or too little of it. It's best to get iodine from food; because of this, we're emphasizing iodine-happy foods in the food categories.

9. Skip the table salt when you can. Don't overdo it.

10. Selenium. This mineral activates thyroid hormones, so you want to boost its levels. It's toxic in large amounts, though, so you only want to take actual supplements if a doctor prescribes them. We'll tell you how to get your selenium naturally.

11. Zinc away. Yet another mineral needed by the thyroid! Go for healthy meats and shellfish.

12. Iron up! Your thyroid's health depends on getting enough iron. As with all minerals and vitamins, get them through food if possible. We'll point out your iron foods as we go.

13. Apportion your portions. Don't eat too much in one sitting—or else. Your blood sugar will spike and then crash. Eat slowly, so you know when you're full.

14. Fast for ten to twelve hours. That is, stop eating after 8:00 p.m., and don't eat breakfast until at least 6:00 a.m. When you're sleeping, your body makes hormones, including thyroid hormones. It draws energy from stored fat to do this, which is great for your overall health.

15. Let's talk gluten. Gluten is a protein in wheat, barley, and rye. In gluten-sensitive people, it can damage the small intestine. If you're allergic or sensitive to it, you won't absorb the nutrients that are important to your thyroid health. Check with a doctor, watch your symptoms, and look at your family history to figure out if you should be gluten-free.

16. Let's also talk low-glycemic and low-carb. But this area is a "just depends." Some people with thyroid issues need to reduce sugars and carbs. A doctor can let you know if this applies to you.

17. Fiber confusion. Some people have thyroid issues that call for a lowering of fiber, which means lay off legumes and veggies. Then again, some thyroid challenges cause struggles with constipation, in which case you need more fiber. Does either scenario apply to you? Check with a professional.

Food Categories

Here we go! Let's examine all the food-type decisions you should focus on.

Proteins: In general, go for healthy proteins, those that are lean and free of chemicals and toxins. Specifically, focus on ionized proteins, which are found in foods like baked fish. Select those rich in omega-3s and selenium, which decrease inflammation. Great choices? Salmon, tuna, sardines, cod, sea bass, halibut, and perch. If you're a meat eater, have at it. All meats are great, including lamb, beef, chicken, duck, and turkey. Go lean, though.

If your thyroid is troubled, limit foods that are high in soy protein, as these can interfere with the absorption of thyroid hormones. Included are edamame, tofu, tempeh, and miso.

Also select gluten-free seeds, such as chia and flax. Brazil nuts are great too due to their high selenium content. Same with macadamia nuts and hazelnuts. Need iron? Opt for cashews, almonds, sunflower seeds, and pumpkin seeds. If you have thyroid challenges, avoid pine nuts and peanuts.

Fats: Your thyroid is hungry for good fats. Try olive oil, avocado, and healthy nut oils. Then there are the omega-3 fatty acids, which are found in oily fish. Want a cooking oil? Choose those with monounsaturated fats, such as canola oil and peanut oil.

Polyunsaturated fats can lower LDL cholesterol. Go for vegetable oils to meet this need, including safflower, sunflower, sesame, and corn oils—but if you have thyroid problems, skip the soybean oil!

Avoid fatty meat fats and trans fats, like partially and fully hydrogenated oils. They'll clog you up.

Carbohydrates: Currently, there are a lot of arguments about how many carbs per day are good for the thyroid. Ask a professional if you should go low, high, or middle range in glycemic levels. No matter what, select whole grains, such as brown rice and whole-grain pastas. If you eat cereal, consider selecting the fortified brands. Beans can give you sustained energy (although if you are supposed to limit fibers, watch it). As we've discussed, consider abstaining from millet and gluten. Then get creative about carb "additives." Shaved, shredded, or grated coconut gives a zing to any dish.

Vegetables and Fruits: Seaweed is your friend. We're serious. Kelp, nori, and wakame are naturally blessed with iodine. Can't quite stomach the seaweed on its own? Toss it in a salad. In fact, try this simple salad:

Blend together dulse and wakame seaweed. Add in some tamari, rice-wine vinegar, and sesame oil. Grate a little ginger over your concoction. Sprinkle lightly with salt and sesame seeds and eat up. You can also add some fresh mint or lime basil.

Because your thyroid is sensitive—sort of like you are, intuitively— there are a lot of Nopes in this category. There are also some foods to "mindfully manage." Overall, watch out for starchy plants like sweet potatoes, cassava, peaches, and strawberries. Limit your cruciferous veggies, which include broccoli, brussels sprouts, turnips, bok choy, kale, spinach, cauliflower, and cabbage. They can block the thyroid's ability to use iodine. If you are going to eat them, cook them first.

Try the nightshade family if you're not sensitive to them. In some people they can cause inflammation and sore joints due to their solanine content. This includes eggplants, tomatoes, and bell peppers. But skip the white potatoes in that family.

Other good choices include zucchini, artichokes and artichoke hearts, bamboo shoots, sugar snap peas, bean sprouts, carrots, beets, hearts of palm, cucumber, radishes, okra, turnips, rutabaga, and most salad greens.

Dairy: Unless you're allergic to dairy, go for it! Milk, cheese, yogurt. We especially like feta or goat cheese for you; it's highly digestible. For yogurt, get a version that is low-to-no-sugar and laden with pre- or probiotics. If you eat eggs, eat both whites and yolks. The whites have protein and the yolks have iodine and selenium.

Liquids: Well, you can always have water. The truth is that coffee, green tea, and alcohol can all irritate your thyroid gland. A good starter goal for water? About eight glasses a day. Then work up to whatever feels comfortable.

Getting bored with water? Okay then. How about throwing in some fruit and herbs? Maybe a slice of pineapple and a sprig of sweet basil? Or try a couple of strawberries and some leaves of chocolate mint in sparkling water. Even lemon in sparkling water will give you a fix and some fizz.

For hot drinks, herbal teas are a great go-to. If you have hyperthyroidism, avoid ashwagandha tea. If you have hypothyroidism, drink lots of it. You can also make your own hot tea by steeping ginger in water, adding fresh lemon juice or lemon, and perhaps dropping in a touch of coconut nectar for sweetness.

Supplements and Spices: As a reminder, skip the table salt, but eat foods that are replete with ionized sodium, such as seaweed, tuna, and eggs. Your thyroid will thank you. And then think Italian seasonings, like basil and oregano. They help flush the body.

As we've told you, the thyroid hungers for minerals like zinc, iron, and selenium, and it's best to get these minerals through food. But if you plan to use supplements, you don't want to overdose, so let your doctor run some tests before you start.

As for vitamins, there are a few you could consider, although, like minerals, food sources are best. Vitamin D deficiency can be linked to the development of autoimmune thyroid issues. To get more of this through your diet, eat your fatty fishes, cereals, cheese, and egg yolks. A lack of vitamin B_{12} can also wreak havoc on your system. Again, try foodstuffs, like the fish and dairy you're eating for vitamin D, or meat and poultry. Is there a supplement you might really want to take? How about probiotics?

The Nopes

Well, we've really covered your Nopes already, so we'll just summarize them here.

- The whites. No white sugar, white flour, white rice, or white potatoes. And no sneaky sugars, like brown or cane, molasses, honey, or the "-oses" on the label, like dextrose and fructose.

- Fatty foods, like butter, meat, and anything fried. Bad fats can interfere with the thyroid's ability to make certain hormones, and if you are on thyroid medicines, they can block the absorption of those medications.

- Packaged and frozen foods. Too much sodium! You need the correct balance of sodium—don't throw off your balance with these high-salt foods.

- Excess or too-low fiber. If your thyroid is low on fiber, getting too much of it from beans, legumes, and veggies can block the absorption of any medications. If it's too high, you'll get constipated.

- Java too early in the day. Are you on thyroid medications or supplements? Take those medications with only water in the morning. Wait about an hour before you go for coffee, as it can block the medications.

- Alcohol. Sorry. The brew—or any type of alcohol, actually—can play havoc on your thyroid hormone levels. Cut it out or be careful.

Of all chakra types, you face the most complications when it comes to putting together a diet plan. So, we'll create menus for two days for you. Try mixing and matching these.

Breakfast choices can include the following:

1. Cherry/berry smoothie: Mix probiotic yogurt or coconut milk and dark cherries and berries. Toss in a handful of spinach for some greens. Need a little sweetener? Test stevia. Sprinkle a few coconut flakes over the top and drink up.

2. Almond butter/chia cup. Mix a tablespoon of unsweetened almond butter and one tablespoon of organic cocoa powder with one cup of milk of choice or a probiotic-rich, unsweetened

yogurt. Add stevia for sweetener if you like. Add three table-spoons of chia seeds and mix together. Top with grated coco-nut shavings or raw cacao nibs.

3. Three-ingredient pancakes: one mashed banana, cinnamon to taste, and two eggs. That's it. Mix it all together and cook it up. Top with fresh berries or a nut butter of your choice. You can also substitute a boiled or baked sweet potato for the banana.

Lunch selections can include these:

1. Mediterranean chopped salad. Choose from the following: spinach or arugula leaves, tomatoes, bell peppers, red onion, cucumber, garbanzo beans, black olives, and goat cheese. Mix and then dress with vinegar, olive oil, and fresh herbs like basil, oregano, or thyme, as well as iodized sea salt and pepper.

2. Salmon "sandwich." Cook the salmon the night before and mix with yogurt or organic, egg-based mayonnaise in the morning. Add veggies to suit and stuff in a gluten-free or whole-grain pocket bread.

Dinner options include:

1. Black beans and rice veggie bowl. Mix black beans and brown rice. Separately, stir-fry selected veggies with avocado or olive oil and combine. Top with some avocado and lemon juice. Season to taste.

2. Buckwheat delight. Buckwheat is often well tolerated. Cook up your buckwheat and mix in goat cheese and stir-fried meat. If you're not a meat eater, that's okay, since buckwheat is actually a complete protein anyway. Separately, sauté kale, kelp, and other types of seaweed, or spinach and spice with garlic and onion.

Want a few fun snacks? Okay, it's fine to do dark chocolate every so often, and dark berries or cherries are great. Maybe dip the berry in melted dark chocolate? Yes, please. And if you need to crunch—because Communicators love to do that—make popcorn. Don't drizzle it with butter. Try garlic and parmesan cheese after splashing a little avocado oil over the popcorn. If you want a sweet rather than savory snack, drizzle with coconut oil and a dusting of cocoa powder.

REAL-LIFE EATING TIPS

How are you going to live as a real-life food nut? Here are a few tips.

Food Prep

You—*alone*—in a kitchen? At best, you'll lose energy after mixing exactly two ingredients. After all, you're a Communicator. Want to create awesome (or at least edible) dishes?

Cook (or chop or even chomp) while chitchatting with a friend in the room or on the phone. Prep with a mate—a friend, a relative, a kid—in the kitchen with you. Play music, podcasts, or audiobooks. Dana even has a friend who turns on a small television in her kitchen to keep her company when cooking.

Let's imagine you get through your culinary prepping duties. Now what? Not a good thing, a Communicator dining alone. Set two places. Put a picture of someone you love across from you. If you're alone, no one is going to know you are talking out loud. P.S.: Pets count, as long as they can sit still for long enough. Which a dog would, if you employ bribery.

If it's a family meal, stoke the conversation with question starters. Write down twenty or so interesting questions you'd like to ask your loved ones. Pop them into a Mason jar and take turns drawing questions out and answering them.

Grocery Shopping

Your incessant desire to chitchat can make you bored in a grocery store. Not good. That only leads to tossing a fancy pie crust or exotic box of crackers into the cart. Make your grocery list with a friend be-fore you show up at the grocery store. Short of that, read labels. You're a Communicator. Use the gift.

Dining Out

Be careful here. Most Communicators love to converse. Opened your mouth to talk? Oh, how did that eclair slip in? You love dining out with others because conversation is assured. However, if you're din-ing alone, go to a place that plays good music or has televisions, or take a book. Decide what to order as soon as you sit down. Eat only what's on your plate. Don't ask for that second glass of wine or dessert as a way to extend the conversation. And keep your fork on your own plate, if someone sits across from you. It's all too tempting to try their food too.

BONUS MATERIAL—BEYOND FOOD

It's not all about food. There are also a bunch of activities that can lead you skipping down the path of health. And here they are.

Exercise and Movement

Given your sometimes-anxious nature, we recommend walking. You can do it fast or slow, but the steadying action will calm you down. Same with kayaking, canoeing, dancing, or anything rhythmic. Want to stay motivated? Get an exercise buddy or talk on the phone while you're moving. And audiobooks and music to motivate you also work well.

Yoga is great as a stress buster for Communicators; the breathing boosts the thyroid.

But what if you have hypothyroidism? Pick up your pace; try flow yoga. Lift weights. Keep off that weight with moderate or high-aerobic activities. Run. Hike. Row. Or walk fast.

Mindfulness and Spiritual Practices

Among all the chakra types, it's most vital for you to gain control of your intuitive gift. You only want to connect with beings that are supportive of your true self, not with any others. To do so, we suggest you use the following exercises, in the order offered.

EXERCISE: GETTING A GATEKEEPER

A Gatekeeper is a being that serves as your main contact to the spirit world. It keeps out the riff-raff, serves as a filtering system, and provides you needed information and healing energies. To get a Gatekeeper, follow these steps.

1. Connect with your inner self and whatever you call the One.
2. Ask for a Gatekeeper, a being appointed by the One to manage all spiritual concerns.
3. Take a few minutes to relate to the being that shows up. What do they appear like? Feel like? Ask them to give you a message, whether in sensory, verbal, or visual form. Request to know their name and ask that they tell you how they'll communicate with you.
4. Gratitude. Thank the Gatekeeper for serving as your guide and guardian, and remember to consult them about any concerns, even what to eat and not eat.

EXERCISE: CLAIRAUDIENCE AND FOOD CHOICES

Want to use your clairaudience to know what food choices to make? You've already obtained a Gatekeeper, so allow them to assist you. While making a food-related decision, from creating a grocery list to picking a menu item and everything in between, simply pause for a few moments. Link with your inner wise one and connect with your Gatekeeper. Request that they clearly tell you what decision to make. You might hear an inner or outer verbal message, receive an image, or just sense a knowing. Thank them and then follow through.

EXERCISE: CLAIRGUSTANCE AND CLAIRALIENCE: YOUR WAY TO A
HEALTHY, HARMONIOUS WEIGHT

How can you get your clear-tasting and clear-smelling abilities to
work for you? The following tips will help:

1. If a good-for-you food isn't appetizing but you know you should
   eat it, connect to spiritual guidance and ask to have the flavor
   transformed into a great taste. Now eat the food as fast as you
   can.
2. Craving something not good for you? Man, it's so unfair when
   everyone else is stuffing their faces with ice cream sundaes or
   vodka gimlets, right? Don't join them. Instead, imagine you are
   joining them. Your clairgustance will kick in.
3. You just have to eat that fattening artery-hardening cupcake,
   right? Wrong. Use your clairalience to make that cupcake smell
   like a rotten tomato. Disaster averted.

Sleep and Relaxation

Sleep and R&R don't necessarily come easy for you. There's a lot on
your mind! Philosophies to ponder, people to connect with, down-
loads to receive—and we don't just mean computer ones. It's hard
to turn down your inclination toward learning, and thus your over-
anxious mind. Solutions? Use a white noise machine. Sing or hum to
yourself. Read yourself to sleep, or listen to a podcast or audiobook.
Guided sleep meditations are a surefire way to have you drifting off
quickly.

Stress-busting and Prevention

There are two sides to your stress-busting coin. First, you *are* a Communicator! So be loud. Converse. Talk with the same friend every
day. Join groups. Exercise with a buddy or join a group class. Go out
for coffee after an intense meeting. Tea dates with friends, even if
they're short, are lifelines.

The other side of the coin? Try quiet. You need to balance the incessant data input with peace and calm. Create a private space in your yard or home in which you can simply sit in silence.

Self-Care Rituals and Needs

You need your own person to talk to, someone who will accept you no matter what. Call them a spiritual advisor, therapist, or coach. Get listened to.

Then use your communication abilities to create or express yourself. Let yourself channel a book or poetry, write your own music, or take singing lessons. Think "expression" and you'll show how you care—for yourself.

SELF-ASSESSMENT QUESTIONS

In order to build your chakra map in part III, you'll want to pick and choose from the concepts and tips provided in this chapter. Spend some time focusing on these questions, and take notes if you can.

1. What's one personal trait that you wish to fully embrace and build on?
2. What's a weakness that you now know to be watchful for?
3. Which foods from the recommended list are your favorites and should be included in your plan?
4. Which foods from the Nopes list do you need to take out of your current diet?
5. What are some possible substitutions for the Nope foods?
6. What do you fear could be the trip-up point, or downfall, of your new plan? Is there a professional or someone you know who could help you with that?
7. Take stock of your current pantry and food items. Are there any items you should toss out so as not to be tempted?
8. What recommended supplements do you already use, or want to start using, to support your health?

9. Which of the quick tips and real-life tips do you want to use?

10. What grocery shopping and dining habits can you change to help you follow your new plan?

And a few extra questions:

1. What are two forms of exercise mentioned for your type that appeal to you?

2. What one mindfulness or relaxation technique can you implement when stressed?

3. How about sleep? Is there a way you can improve it? Can you plan better to dedicate more time to nodding off?

4. Select a self-care ritual you know you'll do.

5. Is there another chakra that you would like to strengthen within yourself? If so, what foods or activities can you implement from that specific type to help bolster that chakra within you?

9

VISUALIZER

Purpose: To Visualize
You live for visions. Visions of beautiful scenery, art, colorful dreams. You dream in stunning colors and inspiring pictures. Likewise, you perceive the big picture while dreaming big—for yourself, members of your family, or even a group of people. In the same vein, you feel and act your best when you're surrounded by a pleasing environment and you like your "look." Guess what? You'll also eat healthiest if you nourish yourself with attractive and visually interesting foods.

Chakra Location: Pituitary
Tiny but powerful, this pea-sized master endocrine gland is located behind the nose, near the underside of the brain. It pumps out hormones that are essential for your body's well-being.

Color: Purple
Purple reflects the qualities of power and heightened spirituality.

Chakra Affirmation:
I am perfect as I am.

VISUALIZER PERSONALITY TRAITS

Hey, Visualizer. You are the chakra type keyed in to aesthetics. Not only do you notice what's right about the things you can see with your eyes, but you also notice what's askew, or weird, or just doesn't belong. You have an eye for design, art, fashion. In fact, you may even be able to see more colors and slight differences in hues than the average human can.

As a Visualizer, you'll love looking your best, and figuring out how to make foodstuff choices with all the bright colors of the rainbow. Get ready to learn all about how best to support your body.

The call to hold and act upon visions is a sacred one. Are you ready to learn more?

WORDS TO DESCRIBE YOUR VISUALIZER SELF:
Curator. Dreamer. Observant. Designer. Perceptive.

Your main intuitive gift is clairvoyance. You have the capacity to "clearly see." Some clairvoyants can see the dead or the future, dream in Technicolor, or even use their x-ray vision to psychically describe what's happening medically in the body.

Perhaps you're more apt to apply this gift psychologically, such as occurs when you're struck with a deep insight about another's motivations or needs. Or you might effortlessly notice another's self-sabotaging pattern. Maybe you picture what's essential about someone, much as Michelangelo did when carving *David*. Then again, maybe you're more practical. Your gift straight-out belongs in the business world, in which you're highly strategic and simply know what lies ahead.

When it comes to food, you'll have an easier time ordering if you can see the food rather than simply reading about it. Your weak spot? Glass cases with rows of cakes and fresh treats. On the plus side, you can easily graze through a salad bar stocked with healthy ingredients. Later in this chapter, we'll provide two exercises designed to help you benefit from this cool gift.

Your major motivator is seeing the big picture. You can see the big picture, but also which small, detailed strokes formulate a grand masterpiece. Because you can imagine an outcome—a final product or far-reaching impact—you can courageously impel yourself to complete creations and realize ideas.

Your hidden fear is that no one will accept you as you are. You're hard on yourself. You may find yourself engaging in negative self-talk or berating mind chatter about how you look or present to others. What you long for is unconditional acceptance. No matter how you look or feel. The trick is learning to accept yourself fully in every moment. To embrace your shadow as well as your light.

Your greatest strength is your sight. Insight, foresight, and hindsight. In all things, you're a visionary. You can hold visions for yourself, but also for those around you—and even for organizations. When combined with integrity, your revelations allow access to your leadership capabilities.

Here are a few notes about these clairvoyant, sight-based capabilities. In short, you are the following:

- Futuristic. You can make smart decisions, because you can imagine what might happen.

- Clear about yesterday. Your hindsight allows you to perceive the nuances of the past. In turn, this knowledge lets you improve any situation, person, or relationship.

- Artistic. You have an eye for aesthetics, be it in art, design, fashion, landscaping, graphic design, or any number of other activities.

- Devoted to beauty. Ahh, your heart swells with gratitude for the people and places that are beautiful. Of course, beauty isn't only skin deep. Everyone is beautiful inside, and you know it.

- Strategic. You are a master of strategy. So—plan, plan, plan.

Your greatest weakness is being too self-focused. Great visions don't always lead toward the highest outcome. Keep an eye (or two) out for these tendencies.

- Misperceptions. Life is complicated. Your insights might not be 100 percent accurate.

- Being stuck in your head. Certain beliefs can get anchored in your brain and distort your ideas. For example, imagine you've decided that *all* sugars are bad. Wait! Fruits are necessary for a healthy system, and they contain sugars. Every so often, it's good to question your basic assumptions.

- Obsessive around aesthetics. Sure, appearances are important. But obsessing over appearances can cause paralysis.

- Poor self-esteem. Guess what happens if you apply your standards for visual perfection to your own body and being? The answer: emotional pain, and sometimes food disorders.

- Overly emotional. It's easy for a Visualizer to allow distorted views to dominate relationships, situations, or other aspects of life. By seeing yourself clearly—with love—you can better navigate this world and make healthier food choices. (That's right. That chocolate cake will *not* make you love yourself better.)

- Narcissistic. You run the risk of dwelling only on yourself. Keep a sense of humor about all things self-related and you'll be more enjoyable to be around and have more joy yourself.

Achieving a harmonious weight. Your right weight is all about your self-image. Technically, there are two wheels on every chakra. The outer wheel holds your negative programs, as well as others' distorted ideas about you. The inner wheel—picture the hole in a donut—is full of your spiritual, accurate self-image. It's easy for you, the Visualizer, to get confused about how you should act, who you should be, or even how you should look! Why? You can dial in to others' visions about you and enter a state of confusion. Be on the lookout for confused energy, specifically around mealtime. Take the next few steps to combat confusion and stay clear on your best food choices. Every time you eat, take a few deep breaths and decide you're going to operate from your inner image. In fact, picture this internal self and keep in mind how healthy this self appears. You'll automatically make food selections that will manifest this awesome self.

Your chakra endocrine gland is your pituitary: you make* all *your food choices with this gland in mind. This pea-sized organ is located in

---

CASE STUDY: ARNE

Arne had been a picky eater since he was a child. "You can only imagine how I struggled to eat my mom's German cooking," he said. "It's all brown!"

Arne was obviously a strong Visualizer. When asked what foods he enjoyed, he stated, "Foods that don't run into each other on the plate."

Arne loved his job as a photographer, though he admitted the projects that featured "dull objects" were much more boring than his landscape or nature assignments. True to form, Arne was all visual, and was already selecting his foods based on his pictorial palate.

your brain, behind the bridge of your nose. It is referred to as the master gland, as it controls the adrenals, ovaries and testes, and thyroid, among other hormones. These hormones keep the body running, healthy, and happy—or not.

In a nutshell, the "choices" of your pituitary gland impact most of the other endocrine glands. This physical task mirrors the sixth chakra's subtle energetic job. In this chakra, you continually make unconscious choices that decide what you'll do based on self-perception. The healthier your self-concept, the healthier your life sections, including those related to food.

FOOD AND SUPPLEMENT PROGRAM FOR THE VISUALIZER

It's time to talk shop—everything from food selections to actual shopping strategies. Let's get going.

Holding Arne's personality as vital, we weren't going to alter his striking attraction to color and beauty or the negative space he desired on his plate; rather, we needed to work through and with it. Arne had a personal goal of "beefing up" so he could feel more attractive, so we kept that in mind too.

Immediately, we helped him create a list of colorful foods to buy. In fact, we recommended that he only buy ingredients he thought were beautiful, so he'd be more apt to cook with them. Then we had him add color to his kitchen so he'd want to spend more time there, in addition to making a list of healthy, organic-based restaurants that were well decorated. Next, we encouraged him to buy a few new items of clothing that would add gusto to his self-image. Arne was also willing to work with a naturopath to

Quick Tips and Tricks for the Visualizer

A quick reference of your big takeaways.

1. Follow a diet replete with fish, eggs, fruits, and nuts. Add in lots of leafy greens and pair carbohydrates with proteins. Maybe check out a ketogenic diet. But go *low* carbs, not *no* carbs.
2. Assess for food allergies and sensitivities. See a physician, endocrinologist, allergist, nutritionist, or naturopath.
3. Go organic and hormone-, pesticide-, and antibiotic-free, as well as free-range and wild-caught. You don't want anything to interfere with your natural hormones.
4. Eat your larger meals for breakfast and lunch and eat dinner at least three hours before you go to bed.
5. The pituitary gland could be considered the brains of your endocrine system. With that in mind, consider some of the science of the hormones the pituitary makes. (Okay, this might get a little boring, but it's all good stuff.)
   - Human growth hormone (HGH) is essential for growth and tissue repair and is produced during sleep. To sustain

formulate the exact right balance of fats, carbs, and proteins for muscular growth, and to join a gym, where he employed a personal trainer to work up a lifting regimen.

Arne was excited and jumped into his new program with little resistance. His weak spots? Beautiful desserts. He agreed to carry organic cocoa products with him, as well as other healthy snacks, to eat instead. Then he adopted our clairvoyant suggestions, stopping to visualize the light—and himself as a light—whenever he was tempted to eat out of bounds. And once a week, he met a friend at a place of sheer beauty, like a local lake, to drink in the sights and fill his soul.

healthy levels, consume melatonin-rich foods, including chicken, pork, salmon, eggs, strawberries, cherries, Chinese wolfberries (also called goji berries), oats, and black, red, and basmati rice.

- Adrenocorticotrophic hormone (ACTH) prods the adrenals to make cortisol. Having too much and too little cortisol are both bad things. To help balance this hormone, avoid alcohol, sugar, and caffeine. On the plus side, it's okay to reach for (some) dark chocolate, pears, and probiotics.

- Luteinizing hormone (LH) and follicle-stimulating hormone (FSH) stimulate the reproductive organs to produce estrogen, progesterone, and testosterone. Aid this by selecting foods with high levels of magnesium. Good choices include spinach, fish, kale, figs, and green beans. Seeds, like pumpkin and roasted squash seeds, hemp, flax, and chia are also fantastic.

- Thyroid-stimulating hormone (TSH) does just what it says. It motivates the thyroid to produce its own hormone: thyroxin. Magnesium, as we mentioned, boosts the thyroid. Selenium, found in nuts like Brazil, macadamia, and hazelnuts, also bolsters your TSH. Iodine too is beneficial. How about seaweeds like kelp, dulse, nori, and wakame? Learn to like these salty seaweeds by adding them to salads and stir-fries—or try Asian wraps and rolls, like sushi.

- Melanocyte-stimulating hormone (MSH) isn't yet well understood, but early research notes it enables skin pigmentation, ultraviolet protection, and more. A deficiency of this hormone can result in high levels of inflammation, chronic pain, and problems with sleeping, as well as heightened appetite and obesity. Low levels can also denote the presence of mold biotoxin, so check with a mold specialist. To support healthy levels of this important hormone, try a cocktail of three supplements simultaneously: liposomal glutathione, non-yeast-based selenium, and dibencozide. (Maybe check out whether you need that cocktail with a professional first!)

6. Get regular, uninterrupted sleep. Hormone production and balance happen when you're asleep. Best case? Go to bed and get up at the same time each day. We know it's hard, but it's worth it.

7. Go for the right sweeteners—in moderation. You want those that don't sky-high your insulin. Instead, choose monk fruit, chicory root, or coconut nectar.

8. Always pair carbohydrates with a protein. You'll feel full for longer, and the combination will help stabilize your blood sugar. Carbs alone will elevate it. That means "yes" to that bowl of oatmeal, but add a couple of tablespoons of almond or sunflower butter.

9. Go organic. In case you overlooked that advice earlier in the list, we're repeating it here.

10. Talk to your doctor about intermittent fasting. This type of fasting involves skipping food—and only drinking water—fourteen to sixteen hours a day and restricting your food window to eight to ten hours. This action can increase your levels of human growth hormone while decreasing your insulin levels, also supporting cellular repair.

11. Stay hydrated. When you're dehydrated, your body struggles to facilitate proper hormone balance. Lemon water and coconut water, with all those good electrolytes, will help.

12. Keep your blood sugar balanced. Avoid refined carbs and sugars that spike insulin. Add in apple cider vinegar, cinnamon, and fenugreek to help balance your blood sugar.

13. Maintain appropriate iron levels. Too much or too little iron can negatively impact your pituitary. Have your levels checked. If they're not optimal, increase or limit your high-iron foods like beef, chicken liver, or canned sardines in oil. Supplement if needed.

14. Let's talk gluten. If you're allergic or sensitive to it, you won't absorb the nutrients that are important to your hormonal health. Check with a doctor, watch your symptoms, and look at your family history to figure out whether you should go gluten-free.

Food Categories

Let's examine all your best food-type decisions.

Proteins: The pituitary needs protein. Proteins provide the amino acids that produce specific hormones, like HSG and insulin, and they also build cells. Go for organic meats, poultry, and fish. Load up on the lamb, beef, bison, turkey, chicken, and wild-caught salmon and tuna. Steer clear of soy protein, since soy can act as a hormone disrupter. Look into collagen as another source of protein. Make sure it's sourced organic and grass-fed. And if you're okay with shellfish, eat some seafood.

Eggs, seeds, nuts: eat them all. If you're a vegetarian or vegan, ensure you're getting all the essential amino acids. Foods that provide everything in one package include quinoa, amaranth, hemp seeds, chia seeds, and nutritional yeast. It's best to eat nuts that are soaked or sprouted.

Since it's best to have a protein with all three main meals—and snacks—plan to do so. Keep cheese, cubes of meat, or already-cooked quinoa in the fridge at all times. Ready to dine on a meal? Eat your protein first, before you get to the carbs. Then you know you'll have enough room in your stomach. Top your foods with chopped almonds, pair nut butters with fruit, and go for Greek yogurt. It has twice the amount of protein as regular yogurts.

Want to enjoy your proteins even more? Go aesthetic. Place your proteins on a bed of arugula topped with a shredded colorful veggie, like carrots. Set pomegranate seeds around the vegetable bed for additional appeal.

Fats: Two-thirds of your brain is made of fat. Docosahexaenoic acid (DHA) to be exact, which is an omega-3 fatty acid. Feed yourself fats and you feed your brain. You must consume omega-3s and omega-6s, as your body can't produce them. Good sources include fatty fish like salmon, tuna, mackerel, and trout. Eggs, chicken, and lamb liver are also good omega superheroes.

Then reach for ghee, or clarified butter, which is packed with vitamins A, D, E, and K_2. All those vitamins? They compose your hormones. Other best-fat friends include coconut oil, avocados, and olive oil.

Ghee is a staple of Indian cuisine. Here's how to make it.

GHEE

We recommend using a stainless steel saucepan for this. Add the butter to the pan and simmer it slowly until the water evaporates and the milk solids turn a pretty brown. Remove the pan from the stove. Cool for about 5 minutes and pour the concoction through a sieve or cheesecloth. The brown solids will remain in the sieve. Keep the liquid in a glass jar and refrigerate. Scoop it out as needed to use as a fat for cooking, or melt and drizzle over your food. Want to bump up the delicious factor? Once you have your ghee, make it into Patti B's Ghee. Here's how: Add 1.5 ounces of cinnamon (or less if desired) to 1 cup of ghee. Drop in a couple of drops (or to taste) of stevia. Put that on a sweet potato and try not to eat it all in one bite.

If you are a vegetarian or vegan and unable to take in healthy fats from fish or mammals, talk to your doctor about supplementing with a DHA algae option.

Minimize your intake of refined vegetable oils like sunflower, soybean, and safflower. They can incite inflammation. If you do have to use vegetable oil, aim for canola or palm.

Carbohydrates: Buckwheat is a good choice. It's also a complete protein and can stabilize blood sugar levels and eliminate excess testosterone. Chickpeas serve up vitamin B_6, which optimizes pro-gesterone levels.

Select whole grains like brown rice and whole-grain pastas. If you eat cereal, ensure it's whole grain. Maybe even go for fortified cereals and pack in those minerals and vitamins. There are vegetable pastas out there now too. Appeal to the eye with a deep green or colorful goldenrod pasta to keep your clairvoyant self feeling happy. Beans like lima, white, and kidney, as well as lentils, can give you sustained energy. Just remember to pair your carbs with a protein.

GO GREEN PITUITARY SMOOTHIE

Like smoothies? They are famous for enabling you to eat—or drink—a lot of healthy ingredients all at once. What a good way to start your day or substitute a meal. This recipe provides lots of pituitary-friendly ingredients in every gulp.

In a blender, create a healthy smoothie by blending the following at high speed for about a minute:

2 cups water or milk of choice
1 tablespoon raw sesame seeds
2 tablespoons hulled hemp

Then add any ingredients you desire from the following list and process on medium speed until smooth:

2 teaspoons chia seeds, almond butter, raw maca powder, raw spirulina, kelp, coconut gratings, or raw cocoa
1 teaspoon coconut or grapeseed oil
Either a banana or 1 cup of any dark berries

Enjoy!

Vegetables and Fruits: Avocados contain tons of B vitamins, magnesium, and potassium. They're also loaded with healthy monounsaturated and saturated fats.

Make leafy greens a staple: microgreens, collards, kale, spinach, beet greens, romaine, arugula, chard, turnips, and mustard greens. If you like eggs for breakfast, try plating them on a bed of arugula with a side of roasted sweet potatoes. Dress with avocado slices, drizzle with olive oil, and sprinkle sesame seeds over all.

Melons, berries, and kiwis will make your pituitary happy. Yes, you can do fruit salad.

Pile on the antioxidants by eating asparagus, cucumbers, cilantro, red cabbage, artichokes, butternut squash, carrots, and red or white onions. Overall, think brightly colored. Of all the chakra types, you're the one who can eat the rainbow. But one note of caution: some Visualizers can't eat nightshades, like eggplant, white potatoes, peppers, and tomatoes, so test those out.

If you're one of those people who has never met a veggie you liked, primarily because they look unappealing to you, dress them up. Create rosebud radishes and grated garnishes. Learn how to form curlicue veggies and twists. If you don't want to spend the time, get a machine that will do this for you. Why can't you eat a plate of mixed veggies in a variety of pleasing shapes?

Dairy: Currently, there's some disagreement in the dairy area. Some experts insist that dairy should be avoided, as it can be a hormone disrupter. Others qualify their recommendations, assuring that dairy is okay as long as you go for organic, grass-fed, and hormone- and antibiotic-free dairy.

We say, trust your body. How does your skin look after you eat dairy? Does your stomach bloat or not? Give up dairy for two weeks minimum and see what changes happen in your body. Then pay attention to what happens when you add it back. Maybe you'll discover you can do cow dairy—or only almond, coconut, or rice. Make sure you test goat dairy too; it's so good for you!

If you get the green light on dairy, always choose organic products. Eggs are great because they have high levels of melatonin. Yogurt with no added sugar—like goat yogurt or kefir—offers up healthy probiotics. Unsweetened almond and Greek yogurt are also good options.

Liquids: Hydration matters. Load up on the water and add lemon. To keep your electrolytes balanced, drink organic coconut water. Don't drink too much, though, as it's high in potassium and can throw off your electrolyte levels. If you struggle to drink enough water, substitute whole frozen strawberries or other fruits for ice cubes. You will add nutrients and flavor while beautifying the water.

Now let's talk caffeine. It's not *all* bad, but limit, limit, limit. Seriously. Limit. Or try green tea, which boosts metabolism and lowers insulin sensitivity. Stinging nettle tea is not only delicious, but it can lower inflammation in addition to boosting the body's nutrients. And while you should limit alcohol, you can drink nearly unlimited amounts of decaffeinated herbal teas.

Supplements and Spices: The pituitary loves vitamins D and E, so ensure you're getting them in your foods. For vitamin D, go for foods like salmon, canned tuna, and eggs—be sure to eat the yolks because that's where the minerals are. Vitamin E (which you need) can be found in kiwi, sunflower seeds, almonds, and broccoli. Always check with your doctor to see where your levels are and if you require supplementation.

Manganese helps you metabolize your nutrients and digest protein. So consume your greens, almonds, pecans, and brown rice. Brown rice also encourages the production of GABA, a neurotransmitter that creates calm and supports good sleep.

Magnesium helps regulate the pituitary gland. Talk to your doctor if you'd like to add this supplement in the form of a liquid, capsule, or even a high-quality lotion. Foods that provide a magnesium power punch include spinach, fish, nuts, and seeds. Zinc promotes estrogen and progesterone balance, and you can get it from sunflower seeds.

Bee pollen is a fun one. It boasts high antioxidants, possibly boosts immunity, is anti-inflammatory, and aids in detoxification. Sprinkle it over your whole-grain cereal or mix it into your smoothies.

Spice up your meals too. Turmeric and black pepper are a super combo. Turmeric is an anti-inflammatory, and black pepper maximizes turmeric's bioavailability. The brain also loves cinnamon, clove, nutmeg, ginger, and cardamom. Like sweets? Use monk fruit. In fact, experiment. What kinds of healthy cookies can you make with coconut oil as your healthy fat, almond flour as the protein, and monk fruit or stevia as the sweetener? Heck, throw in a little tahini (sesame seed paste) for an anti-inflammatory boost. (And mail us some, would you?)

The Nopes

Well, we've really covered your Nopes already, so we'll just summarize them here.

- Sugar. Really, anything that spikes your insulin. When your body is distracted by insulin and processing sugar, it's not focused on other hormones like estrogen, progesterone, and testosterone, among others. Avoid all the fakes too.

- Hormone disruptors. These nasties include animals, fish, and fowl raised with hormones, antibiotics, polychlorinated biphenyls (PCBs), and mercury.

- Nightshades. You might be one of the unlucky Visualizers who must avoid potatoes (although sweet potatoes and yams are usually okay), tomatoes, peppers, okra, tomatillos, and eggplant. How do you know? You'll feel bloated or inflamed the next day. If not, eat these in cautious moderation, as they can still contribute to hormonal imbalance.

- Refined carbs or consuming carbs in isolation. Skip all refined carbs, and always pair your whole-grain carbohydrates with a protein.

- Alcohol. If you must imbibe, do so sparingly and not to the point of drunkenness. It wreaks havoc on your hormones.

REAL-LIFE EATING TIPS

How are you going to take this healthy plan and apply it to real life? Here are a few tips.

Food Prep

Can you dance and chop? Shake your booty and your spices at the same time? Dancing in the kitchen will release those good-feeling endorphins, taking your enjoyment of food prep to new levels. And think about all that joyful energy you'll be infusing into the food.

Cook with the rainbow. You'll excite visual pleasure and increase your nutritional levels. Then plate your dishes in pleasing ways. Serving food in an artistic way employs your aesthetic gifts, and maybe you can wow your friends and family too.

Once all the prepping is done, set the table using nice plates, candles, cloth napkins, and a centerpiece. Healthy food is easier to eat when it looks good.

Grocery Shopping

You may turn over a lot of produce to pick out the prettiest fruits and veggies. Plan time for perfectionism by making a list before you head out—then check it twice. That way, you'll decrease the temptation to simply choose foods based on pretty packaging.

Dining Out

Dress up! Yup, even if you're just heading for a low-key café. You'll select healthier foods if you like your looks. Ahh, the décor and visual vibe of the restaurant can sometimes be more exciting than the food itself.

Be aware of your temptations, though: anything that looks remarkable but is bad for you. Decide what you're going to order before heading to a restaurant. This will lessen your temptations.

BONUS MATERIAL—BEYOND FOOD

There are also activities that can lead you successfully down the path of health. And here they are.

Exercise and Movement

Exercise is important for Visualizers due to its positive impact on neurochemicals. It reduces levels of stress hormones like cortisol and adrenaline, and pumps up production of those natural mood lifters and painkillers: the endorphins.

What motivates you to move? You'll love any exercise if you dress up for it. Really. Be visually on point.

If you're going to the gym, yoga studio, or dance class, wear cool clothing. Perhaps fun new yoga pants or that muscle tank that shows your physique. Work out in front of a mirror so you can check yourself out in action.

If you're headed outdoors, consider the scenery. You'll love running through the trails, around the lake, or along the ocean more than pounding the sidewalks in the city or circling the local track.

Any sport or exercise in which you can track your physical progress will work for you. Why not kick off a new program by taking pictures, and then take more as you go for a comparison?

Mindfulness and Spiritual Practices

The gift of visual intuition is a fun one. Just make sure you're connecting with supportive beings and information. Toward that end, we suggest you use the following exercises, which you can do at any time.

EXERCISE: CONNECTING TO THE LIGHT

Light is purity. When you connect through the energy of light, you circumvent your overly analytical mind and can receive messages aimed at your highest good. To activate your connection to the light, follow these steps.

1. Close your eyes and settle into your body.

2. Bring your awareness to the center of your forehead and visualize pure white light flooding in through the back of your head. Feel it wash through your pituitary gland and flow out through the front of your forehead.

3. Now ask that your inner sage or Higher Power provide a visual message through the light. If images are coming in too fast, ask that they slow down.

4. Gratitude. Thank the source of this inspiration for serving your highest good.

EXERCISE: CLAIRVOYANCE AND FOOD CHOICES

Want to use your clairvoyance to make healthier food choices? First, conduct the preceding exercise, but allow the light to keep running through your sixth chakra. Then focus on a food-related concern. Request that your inner sage or Higher Power provide a visual message that reveals your best decision. You might see an image appear in the light or even read words of instruction. Ask for additional psychic pictures until you seem finished.

Sleep and Relaxation

Sleep and R&R are dependent on your quieting your mind and resting in a soothing, aesthetically pleasing environment. Bedding matters. Choose soothing colors and fabrics. Paint the walls a calming color, like soft yellow, light green, or lavender. Select shades that make you want to take a deep breath.

Guided meditation will silence your mind. Be your own guide as you close your eyes and count fuzzy sheep jumping the fence. Or imagine a soothing voice speaking in your head, describing the cloudless blue sky under which you lie in a green meadow. You can press star decals onto your ceiling and fall asleep under their sparkling shine.

Stress-busting and Prevention

Instant stress-busting occurs when you simply close your eyes. That's right. If you take away visual stimulation, you calm down. Then behind those closed lids imagine activities or connections that bring calm. Picture yourself petting a dog or floating in a pond. Your nervous system can now reset. We also suggest you create a private space in your yard or home where you can simply sit in silence.

Self-Care Rituals and Needs

Self-care will keep you busy! Schedule your haircuts and grooming appointments. Put shopping days on your calendar, and every week or so visit a beautiful space, like a flower garden or museum. Need a pick-me-up? Get a makeover.

When it comes to self-expression, opt for visual journals or therapeutic art classes. Sketch, paint, or collage out your feelings, fears, and pains; seeing them helps you heal them.

SELF-ASSESSMENT QUESTIONS

In order to build your chakra map in part III, you'll want to pick and choose from the concepts and tips provided in this chapter. Spend some time focusing on these questions, and take notes if you can.

1. What's one personal trait that you wish to fully embrace and build on?
2. What's a weakness that you now know to be watchful for?
3. Which foods from the recommended list are your favorites and should be included in your plan?
4. Which foods from the Nopes list do you need to take out of your current diet?
5. What are some possible substitutions for the Nope foods?
6. What do you fear could be the trip-up point, or downfall, of your new plan? Is there a professional or someone you know that could help you with that?

7. Take stock of your current pantry and food items. Are there any items you should toss out, so as not to be tempted?
8. What recommended supplements do you already use, or want to start using, to support your health?
9. Which of the quick tips and real-life tips do you want to use?
10. What grocery shopping and dining habits can you change to help you follow your new plan?

And a few extra questions:

1. What are two forms of exercise mentioned for your type that appeal to you?
2. What one mindfulness or relaxation technique can you implement when stressed?
3. How about sleep? Is there a way you can improve it? Can you plan better to dedicate more time to nodding off?
4. Select a self-care ritual you know you'll do.
5. Is there another chakra that you would like to strengthen within yourself? If so, what foods or activities can you implement from that specific type to help bolster that chakra within you?

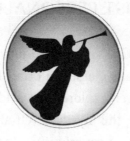

10

SPIRITUALIST

Purpose: Spirituality
You live to connect to a Higher Power and seek relationship with Oneness. Seeking elevated guidance drives you toward higher heights of connection. Want to be healthy? Balance the human with the divine.

Chakra Location: Pineal
The pineal gland, located in the center of the brain, opens the brain to its true potential. The pineal gland produces hormones that regulate mood and sleep, as well as a chemical linked to spiritual experiences, N-dimethyltryptamine (DMT).

Color: White
White reflects the purity and integrity of a life spent serving the Divine.

Chakra Affirmation:
I am living my Divine destiny.

SPIRITUALIST PERSONALITY TRAITS

You are a seeker of spiritual knowledge and yearn to know more. You read, listen, talk, and take classes in order to explore transcendental energies. You may even explore the world of psychedelics in your quest for understanding the mystical. (Or at least read about them.) You'll enjoy altered states of consciousness, namely transcendent ones in which you're connected to the Divine and other spirits.

The call to commune with your Higher Power is a study in self-responsibility. Ready to learn more?

> **WORDS TO DESCRIBE YOUR SPIRITUALIST SELF:**
> Devoted. Ethereal. Reverential. Prayerful. Meditative.
> Philosophical. Aware.

Your main intuitive gift is spiritual empathy. You have the capacity to be aware of the Divine and to treat your body as a receptor for spiritual information. When you're feeling connected, you can sense the spiritual potentials and destinies of those around you. You can also be prophetic. Prophecy involves knowing the destiny of self, others, and even things and places.

It can be easy to tune in to the ego instead of that which is divine, however. When you're linked to a Higher Power, you'll sense peace in your body. To get there, cleanse your self-focused emotions and preferences.

You also have a radar that senses others' honesty and integrity. When someone is lying, you'll know. When they're telling the truth, you'll feel warmer toward them. However, watch your own tendency to tell little white lies in an effort to make life easier for yourself.

As a spiritual empath, you can also develop the ability to perceive clairvoyant images in black, white, and gray in your mind. Black means "no" or "not good for you," white indicates divine approval, and gray indicates an area you're not supposed to look into.

We'll show you how to use your seventh-chakra vision and spiritual empathy to make food choices later in this chapter.

Your major motivator is to commune with your Higher Power. You love seeking unity with your Higher Power. You will read, meditate, listen, and study if these actions aid your understanding of divinity.

Your hidden fear is rejection by the Divine. And that turns into fear of rejection of all kinds. You may react strongly to the feeling of disappointment, which can register as a form of rejection. The antidote? Work on acceptance. Not just of yourself, but of all those around you—no matter the choices they make or the things they do that you may not agree with.

Your greatest strength is your devotion to spirituality. You are a seeker. You want to connect to your own purpose and Higher Power. Because of this, you can easily focus on the following concepts and activities:

- Purpose. You are compelled to discover your life's spiritual purpose. This leads you to work on and improve yourself.

- Meditation. Once you get the hang of it, you can employ meditation to regulate your moods and energy levels.

- Prayer. Want to manifest your purest desires? Find a form of prayer that links your heart to the cosmos.

- Wisdom. When you're balanced, you can apply your wisdom to relationships, career, and health endeavors.

- Acceptance. When spiritually elevated, you possess the ability to accept those who live differently from you.

- Service. Attuned to higher purpose, you know that being of service is the pinnacle expression of humanity.

Your greatest weakness is being egoistic. While your soul longs to connect to your Higher Power, you must remember *you're* not the Higher Power. Sure, you can be connected—but not always to what is best for others. Humility is a spiritual quality, after all. Therefore, watch out for the following tendencies:

- Judgmentalism. If someone doesn't view the world as you do, it can be tempting to consider them wrong. Don't.

- Justification. How easy it is to validate your own opinions, actions, and behaviors when you really ought to accept responsibility for them. Spiritual empathy is not supposed to be a means of "channeling" the Higher Power to back up your personal conclusions.

- Moodiness. If a situation isn't to your liking, your mood could plummet. Work on emotional stability so outside occurrences don't rock you so much.

- Grandiosity. You really don't have all the answers, nor do you need to.

- Spiritual bypassing. This occurs when you hide your psychological or emotional issues or pathologies behind spiritual beliefs. You really do need to deal with your personal issues—they don't disappear behind the veil of spirituality or religion.

- Bossy know-it-all-ness. Yes, you know a lot. Maybe God even talks to you. However, that's not an excuse to be spiritually bossy. That's a recipe for loneliness.

- Overdependence on spiritual connection. You are a human having spiritual experiences. Let yourself be human.

- Masculine/feminine imbalances. Ensure that you are accepting and utilizing your masculine and feminine energies. Your masculine traits involve being active, dominant, and clear. Feminine qualities include being receptive, emotional, and loving.

Achieving a harmonious weight. The Spiritualist can sometimes struggle to hold an energizing weight. On one hand, it can be easy to ignore food in favor of the spiritual high. We know some Spiritualists who spend hours a day meditating, which can make it challenging to work meals and exercise into the day. All that sitting (even if it is for mindful life management) can create a tendency to ignore the physical body. On the other hand, it's tempting to eat away your emotions or uncomfortable spiritual experiences. In addition, a Spiritualist is vulnerable to feeling disconnected—from others and a Higher Power. When this happens, hopelessness can set in which creates a tendency to choose less healthy foods. Ensure you have friends, books, or even a good therapist to help you get reconnected. Then, you'll make your best food choices!

Your chakra endocrine gland is your pineal gland; you should make all your food choices with this gland in mind. The pineal gland is the key to spirituality and so much more. This tiny organ, located in the center of the brain, translates light into messages to run many of the body's chemical processes. For instance, it produces melatonin and serotonin and is key for regulating the circadian rhythms in your body. When it's off, your hormone levels, sleep cycles, and mood get thrown off too.

From a subtle point of view, many energetic factors impact the pineal gland. Think of it as the space for light synthesis. And not just physical light, but the light of higher truths. However, it can also be impacted by shadows, whether your own internal demons or the real ones outside of you. That means that you must be sure you're discerning between heavenly and negative influences. Your ego will have you believe it's always a heavenly influence. Careful.

To keep this chakra pure, prioritize self-awareness. Then take fierce and constant responsibility for your world and your part in relationships. The shadow wins if you justify cruelty or meanness. And watch out for the "Dionysus frenzy" associated with the state of bliss that is sometimes activated by pineal gland highs. Dionysus was the god of ecstasy and spiritual experience in Greek mythology. If you aren't careful, you'll indulge, just like his followers did, in banquets lavish with eggs, cheese, figs, nuts, fish, and wine.

FOOD AND SUPPLEMENT PROGRAM FOR THE SPIRITUALIST

The following quick tips will help you narrow down an eating plan to support your mission of divine connection.

Quick Tips and Tricks for the Spiritualist

1. Go for a balanced diet, focusing on fish and poultry, paired with complex carbs. Round it out with healthy fats and fruits.
2. Assess for food allergies and sensitivities. You can see a physician, endocrinologist, allergist, nutritionist, or naturopath for this purpose.

CASE STUDY: CHENOA

Chenoa believed herself aptly named by her tribal leader. "My name means 'white dove,'" she said. "I've always been a peaceful person."

Chenoa had been raised by her grandmother to follow the Old Ways, and consequently believed in unity among all. She worked for a nonprofit organization and spent much of her time meditating and praying, in the way of her people. She also admitted she wasn't much for bodily movement or exercise, and she'd only focus on healthy foods if someone else cooked her meals—and that wasn't going to happen. However, at her last medical visit, she was warned that something needed to change or she'd be at risk for several serious illnesses later in her life.

3. Go organic and hormone-, pesticide-, and antibiotic-free, as well as free-range and wild-caught.

4. Eat to support your circadian rhythm. The easiest way to accomplish this is to eat your largest meals early in the day and end with the smallest at night.

5. Consider discontinuing any fluoride or synthetic calcium supplements, and avoid chlorine. These can contribute to pineal gland calcification. Want to jump-start this change? Research and follow a pineal gland decalcification detox.

6. You'll be happiest when you eat, exercise, and sleep on a regular schedule.

7. Think of sunlight as a necessary nourishment. Get at least twenty to thirty minutes of sunlight a day and include lots of green plants in your diet. Supplement with vitamin D_3 if needed. Your doctor can do a blood test to double-check your vitamin D levels.

8. Don't be SAD. That's right. The tiny, pinecone-shaped pineal gland can very easily provoke seasonal affective disorder, or

---

First, we introduced Chenoa to her seventh-chakra visual gift. She started to employ her ability to perceive white, gray, and black colors to determine which food choices were good, neutral, or negative. She also began to use this exercise to decide even when to take a walk. She was impressed by how blazing white the "yes" was when she asked.

After a while, she began to notice a pattern underlying many of her food choices. She hadn't recognized her frequent depression nor the fact that she didn't sleep well at night. Depression is often the result of repressed feelings or unmet needs, and Chenoa realized she'd never dealt with the death of her parents when she was ten years old. She entered therapy. As she embraced the deeper sources of her grief, she began sleeping better and felt energized

SAD, which can occur as a bodily response to reduced sun exposure. Called the "winter blues," it can leave you feeling really down and heighten your carb cravings. Combat SAD with exercise, socializing, solid nutrition, and even light therapy.

9. Wake up the natural way. Those blaring alarms aren't your thing. How about using a dawn simulator with full-spectrum light to wake you up gently?

10. Try tryptophan. Found in turkey, salmon, and other foods, this amino acid is converted to serotonin in the brain. To provide serenity, it has to cross the blood-brain barrier. It needs to have carbs to do this, so ingest your meats with at least twenty-five to thirty grams of healthy carbs.

11. Eat melatonin-rich foods. Want a short list? Corn, asparagus, olives, tomatoes, rice, rolled oats, barley, walnuts, flax seeds, pomegranate, and cucumbers.

12. Make friends with alkaline foods. These include chives, cucumber, dandelion greens, onions, parsnips, peppers, okra, lettuce, leeks, pumpkin, sweet potatoes, Swiss chard, and radishes, among others. Alkaline foods support your hormones, as opposed to acidic foods, which cause digestion issues and inflammation.

13. Drink filtered or bottled water. Filter your water through a system that removes the heavy metals, fluoride, and chlorine. Bottled water is also a safe bet. You can also purchase filtered alkaline water or invest in a filtration system.

---

enough to exercise and eat in a healthier way. Deciding to spice up her life, she began taking natural cooking classes, with an emphasis on alkaline foods, and joined a movement class. To compensate for the lack of physical touch in her life, which helped keep her grounded, she began getting massages! In learning how to be cared for by another being, she began to take even better care of herself.

14. If you stare at a computer or television screen at night, invest in a pair of blue light–blocking glasses. They will keep the light from disrupting your hormones and make it easier to get to sleep when it's time.

15. Care for your microbiome. You need the right balance of serotonin in your gut as well as your brain. Load up on pre- and probiotic-rich foods while avoiding artificial sweeteners, refined sugars, and trans fats.

16. Get on board with boron. Boron is a trace mineral that helps decalcify the pineal gland. Foods high in boron include avocados, raisins, prunes, almonds, dates, and hazelnuts. *There's a good excuse to eat all the guacamole.*

17. Sleep. Prioritize undisturbed sleep and aim for seven to nine hours each night. Honor your bed as a place for sleep and sex only.

FOOD CATEGORIES

Here we go! Let's examine all the food-type decisions you should focus on.

Proteins: In general, go for fish and poultry. Make fatty fish a fave. Aim for two portions of salmon per week to boost your serotonin levels. It also provides needed tryptophan and a lot of good brain fats. You can do trout, sardines, and albacore tuna as well.

Chicken, turkey, duck, and goose also make the list of yeses. Avoid frying the meats. Opt instead for baking or grilling. Eggs are another great source of protein and are best prepared boiled, poached, or as an omelet full of healthy greens and veggies. In fact, look back at the alkaline-inducing foods in our tips section and build an omelet using a variety of those. Some people even like salmon- or turkey-enriched omelets.

If you're vegan, get your fill of protein and tryptophan from seeds.

Sesame seeds, chia and flax seeds, cashews, peanuts, and pistachios are high in tryptophan.

Eat proteins high in tryptophan with complex carbohydrates. Why? Most of your serotonin is actually produced in your gut. Tryptophan needs carbs to reach the brain. Nothing wrong with making a whole-grain or gluten-free muffin full of seeds; it would pair perfectly with an omelet.

Fats: To ensure hormonal balance, add medium-chain fatty acids (MCFAs) wherever you can. Try coconut oil, which can be drizzled on just about anything or even ingested by the teaspoon. You can also opt for MCT (medium-chain triglycerides) oil, extracted from coconut oil. But be careful to limit your use to maybe a tablespoon a day. Why? Medium-chain fatty acids head to the liver, causing problems there.

Want to flesh out your fat list? Olive, avocado, and healthy nut oils are super. Canola oil is also healthy for cooking, if you can find a non-processed or cold-pressed version.

While you get the green light for fatty fish, avoid the fatty meats and trans fats, like partially and fully hydrogenated oils. And no lunch meat.

Almonds are a healthy source of fat. As a bonus, they offer lots of magnesium and calcium, minerals that help with sleep. Walnuts are also rich in potassium and folate. Sunflower and hemp are good sources of healthy fats as well as protein.

Want a healthy quick snack you can take with you on the go? Pair seeds with a healthy carb. Our favorite snack mix? Sunflower seeds, either roasted or raw, walnut pieces, dried apples, and dried figs. Drizzle with coconut oil. Sprinkle with cinnamon. Toss into your container and shake. Want a little extra oomph? Roast the mixture for a few minutes before packing it up.

Carbohydrates: Complex carbs are a "yes." They synthesize tryptophan and deliver it straight to the brain, where it increases your serotonin levels. Go for whole grains like brown rice, quinoa, and millet. If you eat bread, opt for whole wheat, rye, or barley.

Kidney, black, white, garbanzo, and pinto beans are complex carbs that also pack in a lot of fiber. Win-win!

Want a healthy treat? Popcorn. And we mean "pop" it—air-popped or stovetop. That way, you can use healthy fats. Then season with grass-fed ghee, which is clarified butter (see page 163 for the recipe). It delivers a healthy K_2 punch. Sprinkle in your own favorite spices to make that popcorn extra special. We like to mix Italian seasoning, rosemary, and pink salt. Mix those into the ghee and then drizzle over your popcorn. You can thank us later. Avoid microwaveable popcorn, as it frequently contains unhealthy trans fats.

Sorry, no refined carbohydrates. They mess with your metabolism, cause inflammation, and can even contribute to insulin resistance. Say no to sugary cereals, white rice, and artificial sweeteners.

Vegetables and Fruits: Think green. Your body (and pineal gland) thrives on veggies and fruits that have been loved up by the sun. Sun-kissed veggies and fruits increase your metabolic energy production. After all, the pineal gland translates light inputs into chemical signals to aid the entire body.

Although fruits can contain simple carbs, they have enough fiber to make them a healthy option. Eat high-fiber fruits like apples, pears, and berries. Bananas contain potassium, magnesium, and tryptophan. Kiwi is a rock star fruit for you, as it contains melatonin, potassium, magnesium, folate, and calcium, as well as antioxidants.

Try spinach, kale, and all sorts of complex carbs, like sweet potatoes and yams. How about beets? They have boron. Chlorella, spirulina, and wheatgrass will cleanse the brain of heavy metals too, which can get in the way of a functional pineal gland. A super healthy, quick meal to get your serotonin cranking? Simmer some sweet potato chunks in veggie or chicken stock until they're tender. Meanwhile, brown some turkey meat (or your favorite meat alternative if you're vegan) that you've seasoned with garlic, onion, and turmeric, and add it to the sweet potatoes. Fix yourself a spinach and kale side salad, adding pears and chia seeds, and drizzle with olive oil. You'll be sighing with ecstasy by the second bite.

For those of you who think your pineal gland needs a little help—as in, you too often feel sluggish, can't sleep, or can't think well—try our pineal gland cleanser.

PINEAL GLAND CLEANSER

Get out your blender. Mix four stalks of kale or spinach leaves, a cucumber, one half of an apple, and a lemon. Drink. Throw in a few walnuts, cacao powder, and stevia if you want some protein. Maybe even do this once a week!

Dairy: Unless you're allergic to certain types of dairy, go for it. Milk, cheese, yogurt. Due to its levels of healthy medium-chain fats, dairy is a helpmate. If you do yogurt, choose low to no sugar and get those brands that are laden with pre- or probiotics. Like eggs? Eat both the whites and yolks; the whites have protein and the yolks have iodine and selenium.

Liquids: Water, water, everywhere. It's great for you. Your best bet is filtered alkaline water. But you can also reach for herbal teas, especially if you add coconut, MCT, or ghee.

Squeeze your own fresh-made juices, going heavier on the veggies than the fruits. It's a great way to get hydrated and fill up on nutrients.

Chamomile tea, especially at night, brings on the snoozes. Why? Maybe it's the flavonoid (plant metabolite) compound it contains, apigenin, which activates gamma-aminobutyric acid (GABA) receptors.

Three warnings: Consider avoiding caffeine. And red wine. And sodas.

About the first piece of advice. Your one exception to the no-caffeine rule? Green tea. It contains compounds and antioxidants that increase metabolic health.

Sodas aren't great because they contain simple carbohydrates, which aren't the best for your system.

Actually, the jury is still out on red wine. If you do pour a glass, keep it to that single one. Alcohol disrupts hormone levels. Also, imbibe at least four to six hours before bedtime. While red wine can make you fall asleep easily, it wakes you up a few hours later.

Supplements and Spices. Although it's best to get your vitamins and minerals from foodstuffs, you may want to consider a multi-mineral supplement that contains potassium, zinc, calcium (not synthetic), copper, and magnesium, especially if you want a good night's sleep. Have your doctor run tests so you don't overdose.

Vitamin D_3 is the vitamin for sun bunnies, which you are. Have your levels checked by your doctor to ensure you're getting enough and that you're absorbing it. Also, consider checking out your folate and vitamin B_6 levels.

Barley grass powder can be sprinkled in your green smoothies. Guess what? It contains tryptophan, zinc, potassium, and magnesium. Green supplements like chlorella, wheatgrass, and spirulina can be helpful, as we've already suggested. And raw cacao helps with oxygenation, while delivering lots of antioxidants.

Apple cider vinegar aids in clearing heavy metals while depositing healthy vitamins, minerals, and enzymes. Your pineal gland will thank you. Add flavor to your food with chives, garlic, onion, turmeric, and cilantro. We also suggest you get familiar with ghee, which we've brought up a few times—with good reason!

The Nopes

Some of these we've already covered, but here's a more complete list.

- The whites. No white sugar, white flour, white rice, and white potatoes. Go super light on sneaky sugars and avoid all fake sugars.

- Excess or too-low fiber. Fiber is important for your gut health, which helps regulate your hormone levels. Too little or too much, and your gut isn't happy.

- Alcohol and nicotine. Both of these can negatively impact your serotonin levels.

- Synthetic calcium. If you're going to take a calcium supplement, do yourself a favor and take an all-natural one. Best bet? Plant-sourced calcium.

- Caffeine. Be wary of caffeine, as it can negatively impact your sleep cycle. If you have caffeine, do so sparingly and always early in the day. (Like we already said, green tea is okay.)

REAL-LIFE EATING TIPS

How can you merge your spiritual self with your human food choices? We have some ideas for you.

Food Prep
Chop, mix, and sauté your organic and naturally sourced food while enjoying high-vibe music or listening to an inspirational spiritual talk. Have a partner, friend, or family member join you in the kitchen and ruminate about God, religion, the Source, or the Divine? Jackpot.

Food prepping is also a great time to bring balance to your sometimes overly spiritual self. Make it a sensual experience by concentrating on the feel of the firm vegetables or the softness of the fish. Remember: you are spiritual, but you're also physical.

Grocery Shopping
Make your grocery list while connected to your Higher Power—in fact, use the exercise found later in the chapter to do just that. Grocery shopping can then be intuitive and quick. Follow the flow of spirit, too, by checking out local growers. Farmer's markets are a stellar option.

Dining Out

Most people consider going out for dinner. But remember, dinner should be your smallest meal of the day. Like restaurants? Try that cozy organic café for breakfast instead.

If you're eating dinner out, try to go somewhere with dim lights and a relaxed vibe to support your circadian rhythm.

BONUS MATERIAL—BEYOND FOOD

There's more to life than food. Here are some other ways to strengthen and nourish your chakra type.

Exercise and Movement

Exercising in daylight helps create order for your circadian rhythms. The morning sun can keep SAD at bay.

Know what else exercise does for you? It helps release tryptophan in the blood while inhibiting other amino acids. And that's the boost in serotonin you need. Aerobic exercise like swimming, jogging, biking, and hiking will get you, and your serotonin, going.

Spiritualists may also like yoga, as it fosters an expanded state of being. Don't skip the *savasana* pose, though. That magical ending pose—also known as corpse pose—stimulates melatonin production.

Mindfulness and Spiritual Practices

You will feel at peace when you feel connected to a power beyond yourself. Use the following exercises to connect with your Higher Power.

EXERCISE: CONNECTING TO YOUR HIGHER POWER

It's easiest to connect with your Higher Power through your higher self, or inner sage. This is the part of you that remains purely connected to the spirit world and resonates with love. Simply follow these steps.

1. Find a quiet space. Sit comfortably and close your eyes.

2. Take a deep breath into your heart space. Feel your breath resonate in your heart. Continue to take deep breaths, then imagine the breath rising to your throat, then up into your forehead.

3. Imagine that your breath continually enters and exits through the top of your head. As you allow this process, ask to connect with your higher self. You may hear a little voice, sense a presence, or feel some emotion.

4. Take a few minutes to relate to your higher self. How does it appear? Ask this self to give you a message in sensory, verbal, or visual form. Then ask it to link you with your Higher Power, and note the beautiful expansion of this Oneness within you. Remain in the love for as long as you desire.

5. When you're finished, allow your breath to fall back into your heart space. Release the sense of your higher self and Higher Power, knowing that the bond will remain.

EXERCISE: YOUR HIGHER POWER AND FOOD CHOICES

Want to use your connective gifts to know what food choices to make? You've already learned to connect to your higher self and Higher Power, so start by running through the previous exercise. Remain linked with your higher self and Higher Power while focusing on a food-related decision. Anything counts, from creating a grocery list to picking a menu item. Request that you clearly receive information on what choices to make. You might even use your spiritual empathy and ask to perceive an image in response to a question, such as "Should I eat X?" Watch as a black, white, or gray vision unfolds. Black is no, white is yes, and gray is a signal to ask more detailed questions. You can use this exercise any time you need to.

Sleep and Relaxation

When we're stressed, the pineal gland hormones are negatively impacted. Then sleep becomes a distant dream. If you feel disconnected from anyone or anything you love, sleep will most certainly elude you. There are solutions. Meditate and pray before bed. If your heart feels heavy, ask your Higher Power to hold it. Consume chamomile tea and inhale lavender essential oil.

If sleeplessness persists, consult with your health care provider about a natural supplement. Perhaps a small dose of melatonin can assist on those fitful nights; just ensure you don't use melatonin for more than three nights in a row or your pineal gland could get a little lazy about making it. You can also try a homeopathic remedy found in your local health food store.

Stress-busting and Prevention

When stressed, you might become anxious, lose hope, judge yourself, and feel disconnected. Yikes! That's quite the cocktail. To bust your stress, spend time reconnecting to your Higher Power. Meditate. Allow silence. Read your spiritual books. Watch videos, movies, and television shows that anchor you in gratitude and connection.

If you're a religious person and belong to a church, temple, mosque, or synagogue, get to a service or engage in prayer.

Self-Care Rituals and Needs

You need uninterrupted time for yourself to commune with your Higher Power. Also allow time to sit in the sun. Soak in all those rays. Close your eyes and feel your body flow into union with all that's around you.

You can also benefit from regular gentle massage. It's good to honor your physical body.

SELF-ASSESSMENT QUESTIONS

In order to build your chakra map in part III, you'll want to pick and choose from the concepts and tips provided in this chapter. Spend some time focusing on these questions, and take notes if you can.

1. What's one personal trait that you wish to fully embrace and build on?
2. What's a weakness that you now know to be watchful for?
3. Which foods from the recommended list are your favorites and should be included in your plan?
4. Which foods from the Nopes list do you need to take out of your current diet?
5. What are some possible substitutions for the Nope foods?
6. What do you fear could be the trip-up point, or downfall, of your new plan? Is there a professional or someone you know who could help you with that?
7. Take stock of your current pantry and food items. Are there any items you should toss out so as not to be tempted?
8. What recommended supplements do you already use, or want to start using, to support your health?
9. Which of the quick tips and real-life tips do you want to use?
10. What grocery shopping and dining habits can you change to help you follow your new plan?

And a few extra questions:

1. What are two forms of exercise mentioned for your type that appeal to you?
2. What one mindfulness or relaxation technique can you implement when stressed?
3. How about sleep? Is there a way you can improve it? Can you plan better to dedicate more time to nodding off?
4. Select a self-care ritual you know you'll do.
5. Is there another chakra that you would like to strengthen within yourself? If so, what foods or activities can you implement from that specific type to help bolster that chakra within you?

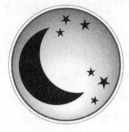

11

MYSTIC

Purpose: Shamanism
You are the shaman of the chakra universe. It's your job to connect the worlds of nature, humankind, and all things spirit. In short, you are a maestro of the mysteries.

Chakra Location: Thymus
Situated in the upper chest, this little-understood gland is all about immunity. It is the eighth chakra's in-body anchor, formally found a few inches above the head.

Color: Black or Silver
There are two basic types of shamans. Which are you? Those described by the color black are experts in power. Are you a silver? Then you're devoted to love. Or perhaps you're a balanced shaman, working equally in power and love. No matter which, you are the priest-healer who links all dimensions and planes.

Chakra Affirmation:
I am free of my past and powerful in my present.

MYSTIC PERSONALITY TRAITS

Navigating so many planes of reality, sometimes you may wonder if you're human at all. Of course you are, but you're able to communicate with the non-human and otherworldly as well. Let's examine all your super personality traits.

Who are you? You're a combination of all the chakra types. You can access all their intuitive gifts and strengths. You can also fall prey to all their pitfalls and weaknesses.

You're complex and magical, so keep in mind that, for simplicity and focus, you'll want to choose one particular chakra type to align your food choices with. That's going to keep your body ticking along and running smoothly. While you may choose to change it up from time to time, you'll need a home-base chakra plan.

> **WORDS TO DESCRIBE YOUR MYSTIC SELF:**
> Multidimensional. Shamanic. Magical. Unusual.
> Mysterious. Enchanting. Otherworldly. Esoteric.
> Mystical. Complex. Deep.

Your main intuitive gift is shamanism. You are a complicated soul. As a Mystic, you can access all the other chakra gifts. That's right. You can access natural, physical, emotional, mental, relational, spiritual, and harmonic empathy, as well as clairaudience and clairvoyance. You can also command forces and walk between all the realms. This mix can cause a muddle. Is a certain feeling your own or another's? Is a physical craving your own or someone else's? You have a lot to keep track of.

Your major motivator is to understand the Mysteries. The term "Mysteries" alludes to secret teachings that explain the origins and functions of the universe. These have been studied in societies across time. Comprehending them is the hidden desire of all Mystics.

Your hidden fear is of unleashing your mystical powers. This fear may stem from subconscious fears of being thought weird or different, or of being excluded. You may be clinging to a mundane way of life as a reaction to your fear of the magical. Our advice? Go full wild. Jump feetfirst into mystical exploration. You can always reclaim the "normal." But how many people have the opportunity to be magical? Feel your fear, and then do it anyway.

Your greatest strength is your otherworldly connectivity. A flick of your finger, wander of your mind, or inspiration from your imagination, and you're off to a different dimension. Think of how many super-wild astral beings are available in these otherworldly planes. You have countless sources of help and assistance in the invisible realm. We'll list just a few of the positives your invisible networking abilities will afford you.

- Healing powers. Spiritual guides are available to send incredible healing energies to and through you. You can connect with the healing essence of a plant or herbal medicine. Then again, you can also bond with an Archangel, deceased ancestor, power animal, or any other spirit being that will share with you insights and offer healing assistance.

- Guidance. Have a question? Among the infinite beings floating around, one is sure to have an answer.

- Perceptivity. You have access to unlimited planes of existence. You're the person who sees the light when others only perceive the shadows. You're also the person who recognizes the darkness where others only see the light.

- Innovative. Among your invisible helpers, one is sure to help you create a new approach to an old problem.

Your greatest weakness is temptation. Your access to, and ability to direct, spiritual beings and powers introduce many temptations.

- Acquiescence to pressure. Many addictions, compulsions, negative thoughts, and awful behaviors are influenced by the hidden world. It's imperative that you be clear about your sources of insight and whose motivations you're following. The exercise "Spiritual Guidance for Food Choices and Cravings" will help you connect to a helpful source of guidance to eradicate a craving and select a beneficial food item.

- Physical stressors. It's one thing to consult with otherworldly beings. It's another to invite their energies into your body or have them manage your relationships. It's physically challenging on your endocrine organs to serve so many energies. The mental and material strain can lead to all the compulsions linked to the various chakra types.

- Susceptibility to the Dark Arts. You can not only cast spells, but also be victimized by them. Engaging your power with malintent or anger will leave you feeling shameful and bad about yourself. The result? You'll treat yourself poorly, including making poor food choices.

- Loss of subtle energies. You are a priest-healer, a spiritual medium who can help others heal. Your drive to help could cause you to give away your own beneficial energies, weakening your powers and related endocrine glands. Then come the food cravings.

- Theft of subtle energies. What you can give, you can take. A little tired? Why not steal someone else's fiery energy? What a boost! Emotionally deflated? Why not borrow some of that happy person's joy? Because you can't process energies that aren't your own. Other people's subtle energies can turn into disease and hardship in your system, even if they create a temporary boost.

Achieving a harmonious weight. Up and down. Thick and thin. The weight of most shamans alters with the particular chakra they are engaging with. Feeling low? On come the second-chakra cravings for carbs in the form of cakes and cookies. Overworking? Someone needs to hide the third-chakra indulgence—popcorn—from you. Feeling bad about the cause you work for (or lack of one)? You'll stop eating. You don't have a weight issue. You have a chakra issue. What do you do? Pick a chakra (more on that later) and stay with it. Pay attention to feeling disconnected from your own body. Mystics are vulnerable to disembodiment. After all, it can feel overwhelming to feel feelings, thoughts, and pains that aren't your own. It becomes second nature to mentally check out of your own body and explore other dimensions and realities. For your own health, ensure that you're dialed into your chosen main chakra and connected to your body before making food choices.

Your chakra endocrine gland is your thymus gland. Make all your food choices with this gland in mind. As a Mystic, your endocrine gland is your thymus. The thymus sits in the upper chest. Biologically, the thymus is one of the two main immune system organs, producing cells that defend the body against all sorts of physical invaders,

CASE STUDY: JAMES

James had been through three different treatment centers when he was younger and was a devotee of Alcoholics Anonymous. He shared that his meetings helped him manage his cravings for "just about everything bad," from caffeine to alcohol to opioids, but did little in the way of dealing with his "fluctuations."

When unpacking the term "fluctuations," James outlined a list of sensitivities, like intense feelings that didn't make sense (because they weren't his), hearing voices in the night, receiving futuristic nightmares, and being aware of the presence of otherworldly spirits. His ability to sense others' physical ailments in his own body was especially troubling, as he was a medic and was constantly around others who were in pain.

including deadly microbes like bacteria, viruses, fungus, and cancer. Once the T-cells, a form of the white blood cell, migrate to the thymus from the bone marrow, the thymus trains and develops them to fight intruders.

The thymus also produces thymosin, which stimulates lymphocytes in other lymphatic organs. So, essentially, the thymus helps clear and clean the trash from your body.

Traditionally, science has believed that the thymus is only active until puberty, even disappearing altogether around age sixty-five. Weird, right? That's why elderly people have less vigilant immune systems. But that idea is now being questioned, and various supplements and treatments have been developed to stimulate the thymus during adulthood.

FOOD AND SUPPLEMENT PROGRAM FOR THE MYSTIC

The foundations for your chakra map will be found in this section.

James was clearly an eighth chakra Mystic. He was loaded with all the intuitive gifts and also burdened by each chakra's weaknesses.

It was vital that James get control of his intuitive boundaries. He enrolled in an intuitive class focused on techniques for identifying and keeping out others' energies; he also read Cyndi's book *Energetic Boundaries*. We then prompted him to select a guiding chakra. Since he worked in the medical field, a first-chakra life-and-death undertaking, he selected the first chakra. Then he began building a plan formatted around the first chakra, Manifestor-type philosophies.

He started building an action plan immediately. Since he already belonged to a gym, he now went for regular workouts. He

Quick Tips and Tricks for the Mystic

Our very first tip is the most important. Embrace it. We've both experienced our Mystic abilities and can testify to their credibility.

1. Pick a chakra and lead with it to make most of your food choices. Really. Every one of your chakras is strong. That can muddle your tastes. Depending on what you're up to, or who you're with, your tastes could duplicate those of another (whether they're dead or alive). That makes it super hard to follow a food program and even harder to ignore the cravings.
   We'll give you an example.
   Imagine you just used your seventh chakra while spiritually relating to a loved one. Seventh-chakra people like fish and broccoli, and (we're stretching here) angel food cake. *Wow*, you think at snack time, *I'll eat cake!* So you do. An hour later, you're dining out with a ninth-chakra sort who follows the Garden of Eden diet, which mainly consists of fruits and veggies. You consume lots of raw food. Your stomach feels upset afterward.

---

also made sure to always have on hand groceries that could be combined for a balance of proteins, fats, and carbs. He set reminders on his phone so he would remember to eat more often. Working with a naturopath, he supported his thymus. And he began deeper mystical training with a local shaman. At first he thought it weird, but his training quickly became his favorite part of the week.

James committed to look up his cravings using our "Mystic Craving Desires and Substitutes" chart so he could find substitutes for unhealthy desires. Then he decided to do something fun once a week and take some time off each year. Following the Manifestor choice, he started hiking in area parks for fun and exploring longer spiritual hikes around the world.

Later you're ready for a bedtime snack, and your partner is a first-chakra meat eater. Before bed, you chomp down an entire steak.

What kind of diet is that? A crazy one! For your overall diet plan, you'll want to select a chakra type and follow its diet.

2. Stop now. Select a main chakra, just in case you haven't. Return to the quiz you took in chapter 2 and follow the directives.

3. Before creating a food program, check for food allergies and sensitivities. Consult a physician, endocrinologist, allergist, nutritionist, or naturopath if you need to.

4. Cleanse. When struggling with cravings, employ the "shamanic cleanse." Eliminate salt, red meat, sugar, alcohol, caffeine, white flour, and dairy products. Eat orange potatoes like yams or sweet potatoes, chicken and fish, and plenty of greens. If you're vegan, choose full-protein grains, such as hemp or quinoa, and eat nuts and seeds. Use healthy fats like the ones we listed under the "Fats" section. After a week on this diet, gradually add back in foods and see how they make you feel. Continue forward only with those that support and agree with you.

5. Overall suggestion. Go organic and hormone-, pesticide-, and antibiotic-free. Then select free-range and wild-caught. While you're at it, the immune system can also be sensitive to MSG, gluten, dairy, GMOs, dyes and chemical additives, and all sugars and fake sugars. As a Mystic, your body is your instrument. Keep it clean and happy.

Now for a few bewares:

1. Beware of entity eating. What's that? You're a shaman. As we've shared, you're susceptible to the cravings of any person or spirit in your presence. At a single meal, you might go for a muffin

because dead Aunt Bethany liked them; tiramisu because of long-dead, never-even-met Great-Grandpa Lorenzo's love of the dessert; and maybe vegan chili because that's what your dining partner likes. That's a diet that will overwhelm, not nurture, your body.

2. Beware of the many chakra-based compulsions. Because you so easily flow from chakra to chakra, so do your moods—and addictive tendencies. Again, stick with a single chakra and you'll at least limit your cravings to those related to that chakra.

3. Beware of "ceremonial" temptations. What does this mean? Shamans around the world are known for entering an altered state to connect with other worlds. They often use ceremonial substances or sacred medicines to accomplish this task. Even if you don't practice shamanism professionally, your soul can easily shift into a trance state, which could unconsciously prompt you to reach for unhealthy substances. In other words, a Mystic is easily tempted to use dangerous substances to get a high. Because of that, we'll list a few of the most common shamanic temptations and healthy substitutes under the "Nopes" category.

4. Beware of ego eating. Shamanic sorts can often transmute energies, turning them from unhealthy into healthy. But do you *really* think you can transform thick-crust pizza into something that resembles fruit, or neutralize soda pop?

FOOD CATEGORIES

We're going to examine the foods you should focus on.

Proteins: You'll want to interweave supportive thymus protein choices with your leading chakra ideas. If you eat meat, go for lamb and organic chicken or turkey. If you select beef, select grass-fed. Eggs are terrific for boosting the immune system, as are wild, fatty fish high in omega-3s, like salmon, mackerel, and others.

Not a meat eater? It's okay. Even if you are, there are lots of options besides meat. Go seeds and nuts. Deserving of praise for boosting immunity are almonds, Brazil nuts, pine nuts, pistachios, walnuts, and pumpkin and sunflower seeds. These selections basically up your vitamin E and selenium. You can also go for mung beans and other legumes.

Fats: In addition to the fats best for your selected chakra, the majority of your dietary fats should be monounsaturated, which are also called oleic, or omega-9, fats. It's said to raise "good" HDL cholesterol and lower "bad" LDL cholesterol, but it also improves immunity. In total, a great list includes macadamia nut, grape, olive, and avocado oils. Coconut oil is a middle-chain oil, but good to use too.

Carbohydrates: First, a warning. Refined carbs, like sugar and flour, turn omega-6 fats (such as those found in meat, soybeans, corn, and other products) into inflammatory chemicals. So stay away. Follow the carb list of your chosen chakra type, but remember to select mainly whole grains, such as brown rice and whole pastas. Rye has been shown to support the thymus too. Beans give lots of sustained energy. In particular, Mystics respond well to root carbs like sweet potatoes, yams, rutabagas, turnips, and carrots.

Vegetables and Fruits: In addition to eating for your chosen chakra type, add five to seven servings a day of vitamin C–rich veggies and fruits. They protect the thymus gland from damage. Include dark leafy veggies, brussels sprouts, collard greens, bell peppers, and broccoli, as well as cauliflower and cabbage. The last three contain glucosinolates, which can protect and enhance the thymus gland. Your thymus gland loves garlic and onions such as shallots, leeks, and chives, so add those to your dishes. Also go for citrusy fruits like tomatoes, berries, and kiwi. For non-citrus fruits try papaya, strawberries, pineapple, cantaloupe, raspberries, cranberries, blueberries, and watermelon. And don't forget dates. They make for a yummy, non-sugary sweet snack replete with vitamins and minerals.

Want to try a great recipe emphasizing glucosinolates, with a dash of protein? Try the following.

PURPLE CAULIFLOWER SALAD

Preheat the oven to 325° F. Cut up a head of purple cauliflower, ¼ head of white cauliflower, and ¼ head of broccoli into medium-sized chunks. Spread them onto a cookie sheet and drizzle with olive or avocado oil. Add salt and pepper to taste, as well as any other spice or herb you like, like garlic powder or chives. Roast for 20 minutes, stirring once or twice. Set aside and cool. If you want, use the cookie sheet again. Drizzle with coconut oil and add grated coconut shavings and almond slices. Roast for a few minutes, until light brown.

Now make a dressing. Consider blending ½ cup of orange or pineapple juice, or a mix of both, along with 2 tablespoons of lemon juice. Add 2 teaspoons of avocado or olive oil and a little salt and pepper. Place the roasted-vegetable mixture in a bowl. If you're a meat eater, you can always add pulled chicken roasted with lemon. Dowse the salad with the dressing and enjoy.

Dairy: For most Mystics, eggs are great. Milk and other dairy products? See how they make you feel. Cow dairy in particular can be very inflammatory, although a sugar-free probiotic yogurt might suit you just fine. Sometimes advised: kefir and ghee. The latter is a highly clarified butter used in traditional South Asian cooking (see page 163 for how to make it yourself).

Liquids: Water. Water. Water. But if you get bored, add a spritz of lime, lemon, cucumber, or orange. Then again, you're a shaman, you can choose from a medley of liquids that can have medicinal effects. Take a walk through the chart "Mystic Craving Desires and Substitutes" under "Nopes." You'll find lots of super liquids to employ, especially if you're struck by specific cravings.

You can also do herbal teas; dandelion root is a good choice. Try white or green teas too. Typically, white teas have less caffeine than green teas, but green teas take the win for healing properties.

Supplements and Spices: There are lots of super supplements and spices that boost the thymus and overall immune system. We'll first list those easiest to obtain.

Echinacea, rosehips, and olive oil. Yup, you can drink olive oil with a spoon. (Not lots of it; just a couple of spoonfuls a day.) Then search for astragalus, black elderberry, curcumin, and oregano oil extract. Beta-glucan is found in the cellular walls of yeast and medicinal mushrooms like maitake, shiitake, reishi, and cordyceps. Beta-glucan boosts the immune system and lowers cholesterol. Take probiotics; much of the immune system is in the gut, and you might as well give your thymus some help. The overarching immune system is fortified by supplements or spices including zinc, garlic, turmeric, and cacao. In Ayurvedic medicine, Indian gooseberry, which is high in vitamin C, tops your thymus list.

Experiments are being conducted using extracts from calf thymus to stimulate thymus growth. Work with a doctor if this approach interests you.

The Nopes

Now for your Nopes.

You have it hard. You need to pay attention to the Nopes of your lead chakra *and* be aware of your tendency toward temptation. Because of that, the following chart will list the most common Mystic cravings and explain the desires underlying them. We'll then give you plenty of healthy substitutes.

MYSTIC CRAVING DESIRES AND SUBSTITUTES

MYSTIC CRAVING	TRUE DESIRE	SUBSTITUTES
SUGAR	Achieve bonding and love; heal old wounds for self or others	*PROTEINS*: Fish or chicken, black or brown beans, seeds and nuts, and other low-fat proteins *CARBOHYDRATES*: Yams and sweet potatoes *VEGGIES*: Greens and cruciferous veggies *FRUITS*: Pineapple, papaya, mangoes, coconut, lemons, and apricots *LIQUIDS*: Cleansing liquids, including alkaline water and red tea, when extra energy is needed

Mystic Craving	True Desire	Substitutes
COFFEE	Boost the nervous system; release negative energies	*Liquids*: To boost the nervous system, drink plain green tea. To detoxify negative entities and energies, use tinctures and teas made from pink yarrow, green tea with lemongrass or mint, or strong black tea. You can also flavor water with fruits or veggies.
TOBACCO	Open otherworldly portals; summon positive spirits; cleanse dark spirits	*Spices*: To open doorways or invite in positive spirits, use cayenne pepper or unsweetened, organic cacao. You can also make a mixture of organic cacao, coconut water, and honey. *Liquids*: Clean dark energy with strong black tea or yellow yarrow tincture or teas.
CHOCOLATE	Ignite clairvoyance; ground the body into the earth	*Spices*: For vision, eat or drink (alone or in combination) unsweetened, organic cacao, ginger, cinnamon, cloves, or nutmeg. *Liquids*: Teas or tinctures of white yarrow help open the third eye. *Carbohydrates and fruits*: To ground, employ cacao with any baked grounding fruits or carbs, such as apples or yams.

Mystic Craving	True Desire	Substitutes
ALCOHOL	Free self from restrictions; summon dark spirits so they can be released or redirected	*LIQUIDS*: For freedom, drink unsweetened, organic red grape or cherry juice. *FRUIT*: To free dark spirits, drink or eat concoctions of dark berries with unsweetened, organic cocoa.
WHITE/ GLUTENOUS FLOUR	Soothe an overly excited nervous system; hiding self from spirits	*CARBOHYDRATES*: To provide comfort, eat carbs approved for your chosen chakra type. *EXERCISES*: To hide from spirits, learn how to use your gifts well, rather than avoid them. Every chakra type features an intuitive ability and an exercise you can employ to develop your aptitudes.
HALLUCINOGENS	Open perceptions of invisible beings; invite light or dark spirits to interact	*SPICES*: For either purpose, go for aromatic spices and tinctures or unsweetened, organic cacao. *LIQUIDS*: Try lightly fermented juices or apple juice with lemon and cinnamon.

REAL-LIFE EATING TIPS

You'll follow the eating tips in your lead chakra description, but here are some extra ones to assure your Mystic self gets things right.

Food Prep

Use your talent. Summon help. A grandmother who died with all the family recipes in her head? She might just help you out. Then again, there are spirits of any nature that can assist. Not yet connected to your invisible helper-beings? Consult your chosen chakra type and follow that food prep advice.

Grocery Shopping

Your Mystic's head can be so high in the sky that getting your feet into a grocery store can be a real chore. Get help. Not only the human type, which will cost you money, but the spirit staff, which is free.

Did your deceased grandmother make the most delicious veggie soup? Ask her to come with you to the grocery store and influence your choice of ingredients to purchase. You may not know why you're reaching for the celery bunch and the yellow onions, but your grandmother does!

Dining Out

Oh boy. Eating out can be a complicated affair. Know why? You so easily adapt to others' chakra types. When dining with a first-chakra person, you might order steak along with them—even though you'd like to be a vegan. Your second-chakra friend is overdoing the french fries because they're feeling emotional? You might end up eating more fries than they do. Remain true to your selected chakra, no matter who you're with, and you'll make better food choices.

BONUS MATERIAL—BEYOND FOOD

Even Mystics have to move their bodies, minds, and souls in practical ways. Add these suggestions to those found in your lead chakra profile.

Exercise and Movement

As a shaman, you live between two—or more—worlds, and you must exercise accordingly. Select exercises that develop your long and short muscles and also deliver anaerobic and aerobic benefits.

Long muscles create elasticity and suppleness. Think of the need to slink around the corners between worlds. Short muscles build up bulk and strength, needed to wield power against adversity. Long-muscle exercises include stretching, yoga, Pilates, and tai chi. Short muscles develop through weightlifting or heavy outdoor work. You can cycle through these types of activities during the week, perhaps rotating a long-muscle exercise with a short-muscle one.

You can also divide your workout times according to anaerobic versus aerobic exercises. Anaerobic workouts (like weightlifting, calisthenics, and isometrics) tear muscle down, requiring the body to rebuild to develop Herculean might. Aerobic exercises (like running, walking, swimming, and dancing) promote cardiovascular health and endurance. There isn't always a neat divide between long muscle and short muscle and anaerobic and aerobic, so try different combinations until you feel happy; then maybe switch it up, so you remain interested in exercising.

Mindfulness and Spiritual Practices

Your life is all about conducting spiritual practices, whether you're awake, dreaming, or in a meditative trance. The "Journeying for a Purpose" exercise will help you perform a journey, a common shamanic practice. The second exercise will ensure that you make healthy food choices and fight off cravings.

Exercise: Journeying for a Purpose

Shamans conduct journeys. Journeys are defined as travels, conducted by the soul, to realms that hold answers or healing energies. Here is an easy and safe way to spiritually journey. Note that some shamans like to have a steady drumbeat to assist in their travel. You can download a shamanic drumming beat from the Internet if you desire.

1. Set an intention by deciding what assistance to receive.
2. Connect with your wise, inner shaman or the Spirit.
3. Request that your consciousness be taken to the site that holds the information, healing frequencies, or connections you require.
4. Remain in that place and stay for as long as you like. Enjoy any exchange of information and energies.
5. Allow the guidance to return you to your everyday state when you're ready.

Exercise: Spiritual Guidance for Food Choices and Cravings

The invisible help available to Mystics can help you make a healthy food choice or resist a craving. Simply follow these steps:

1. Call upon your wise self or the Spirit.
2. Focus on your desire for food. You might have a specific foodstuff in mind or a desire to know what to buy, order, or eat.
3. Ask to be shown the food you should choose. You might sense, visualize, or be verbally given the answer.
4. If you're already focused on a particular food item, request insight about the correctness of that choice. If it's psychically revealed that it isn't healthy, ask for guidance on one or both of these insights:

   The deeper need you're trying to meet with this craving. (Once you understand it, commit to working through the issues involved.)

A substitute food or activity to neutralize the compulsion. (Promise to follow through.)

5. Act on the guidance, and know that you can return to this exercise any time you need to.

Sleep and Relaxation

Sleep can be a rare commodity for a Mystic, especially since your spiritual capabilities are activated at night. You might be so busy visiting with spirits that you forget to sleep.

But you need sleep. All humans do. Conduct your soul journeys, which you were shown how to do in the last category, during non-sleeping hours. You can also ask that the Spirit appoint a spiritual guardian to your body at times you want to relax or sleep.

Stress-busting and Prevention

Above all else, you require subtle energy protection in the form of energetic boundaries. This will keep harmful energies or entities out of your body, mind, and soul. The easiest way to accomplish this goal is to visualize your entire body surrounded by rose, gold, or white energies. If you're feeling really stressed or vulnerable, picture tiny silver mirrors sprinkled throughout every part of your auric field. Each is directed upward. These mirrors will deflect negativity and allow in loving energies.

Self-Care Rituals and Needs

Given your tendency to give away your own good energy and take on others' wounded energies, you owe yourself a lot of self-care. We suggest that every week you pick an activity from the following list. (Hint: These actions each relate to a chakra. By attending to each of the chakras, you address all your needs.)

Physical (Manifestor): Select a fun physical adventure and schedule it into your week. The action must let you blow off steam. This could be hiking, skiing, trail running, swimming, or exploring a new town on foot.

Emotional (Creator): Focus for a few minutes on each of your five feelings: fear, sadness, disgust, anger, and joy. Sense what each offers you while you picture white light clearing it out of you.

Mental (Thinker): Ask your guides to reveal the negative belief causing you the most harm. Replace it with a supportive, truthful one. Keep this new belief uppermost in your thoughts for at least a day.

Relational (Relater): Get in touch with a really good friend. Laugh, cry, play, catch up. Be real.

Communicative (Communicator): Ask your guides to send you an important message—one that reveals a life mystery. Then further research or meditate upon that idea.

Visual (Visualizer): A picture can be worth a thousand words. Request that your guidance gift you a dream or a vision of great meaning.

Spiritual (Spiritualist): Sit quietly and spend time asking to feel the breath, hand, or touch of the Spirit. Then acknowledge that you are worthy of this contact.

Symbology (Harmonizer): Request knowledge of a symbol to concentrate on, one that will bring about great insights.

Natural (Naturalist): Get outdoors! Spend as much time as you can during the selected day playing in the environment. Garden, hike, mountain climb—do anything outside!

Forceful (Commander): Think of something you'd like to command to occur. When aligned with the Spirit's will, go ahead and ask for it to happen.

SELF-ASSESSMENT QUESTIONS

In order to build your chakra map in part III, you'll want to pick and choose from the concepts and tips provided in this chapter. Spend some time focusing on these questions, and take notes if you can.

1. What's one personal trait that you wish to fully embrace and build on?
2. What's a weakness that you now know to be watchful for?
3. Which foods from the recommended list are your favorites, and should be included in your plan?
4. Which foods from the Nopes list do you need to take out of your current diet?
5. What are some possible substitutions for the Nope foods?
6. What do you fear could be the trip-up point, or downfall, of your new plan? Is there a professional or someone you know who could help you with that?
7. Take stock of your current pantry and food items. Are there any items you should toss out so as not to be tempted?
8. What recommended supplements do you already use, or want to start using, to support your health?
9. Which of the quick tips and real-life tips do you want to engage in?
10. What grocery shopping and dining habits can you change to help you follow your new plan?

And a few extra questions:

1. What are two forms of exercise mentioned for your type that appeal to you?
2. What one mindfulness or relaxation technique can you implement when stressed?
3. How about sleep? Is there a way you can improve it? Can you plan better to dedicate more time to nodding off?
4. Select a self-care ritual you know you'll do.
5. Is there another chakra that you would like to strengthen within yourself? If so, what foods or activities can you implement from that specific type to help bolster that chakra within you?

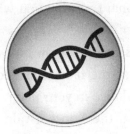

12

HARMONIZER

Purpose: To Harmonize
For you, it's all about harmony and meaning. You find purpose in activism and idealism. What's your cause, your "do or die"? Know that and you'll make great decisions.

Chakra Location: Diaphragm
The diaphragm is located just below the lungs and the heart. When this muscle contracts, your chest cavity expands and fills with air. When it relaxes, air is expelled from your lungs. Your foodstuff choices must support the diaphragm and lungs.

Color: Gold
Gold is the color of enlightenment and divine protection. Always, it indicates an inclination toward the highest good.

Chakra Affirmation:
I embody harmony and peace and bring them with me wherever I go.

You'll only engage in an activity that contributes to a cause. For example, food gardening can be a joy, but only if you can donate some of the produce to a soup kitchen. Likewise, intuitive endeavors and metaphysics will interest you *if* these gifts make the world a better place.

We'll show you how to make foodstuff choices that support your health—and the world's health.

HARMONIZER PERSONALITY TRAITS

The call to bring peace to yourself, your loved ones, and your world is multifaceted. Ready to learn more?

> **WORDS TO DESCRIBE YOUR HARMONIZER SELF:**
> Worldly minded. Activist. Purpose driven.
> Fervent. Impassioned. Zealous. Cause motivated.
> Philanthropist. Moral.

Your main intuitive gift is symbology. Through your subtle senses, you can perceive the healing power of symbols—an uncommon ability. Think hieroglyphics and runes.

You might see a symbol and get struck with a feeling about it. You might visualize a shape and inexplicably understand what properties it carries. Symbols might be formed from shapes, colors, numbers, or other elements. Ultimately, you intuitively know which symbols can bring about healing or manifesting for yourself or others.

Later in this chapter, we'll provide two exercises for opening and applying your gift of symbology to create a better life and optimal health.

Your major motivator is to serve. You love causes and activism. You rev up when it comes to foundations, charities, philanthropy, and just about anything that is "right." If something doesn't feel right? You'll consult your moral compass and put everything in its correct place.

Your hidden fear is that you will be unable to make a difference. You desire to change the world, and the sense that it is your destiny, is so strong within you that the thought that you may not be able to terrifies and paralyzes you at times. Baby steps. Go slow. You'll do it all right, as long as you stay focused and committed. Just one step at a time.

Your greatest strength is your commitment to a cause. As we've shared, you are a philanthropist, an activist, and a cause seeker. You side with the underdog and support those in need. You're more than that, though. You also display the following qualities:

- Purposefulness. You won't rest until you are connected to—and acting upon—your higher purpose.
- Protection. Animals. The hungry. The environment. The abused. You protect what you love.
- Commitment. When you believe in something, you back up your words with action.
- Fundraising. When you're devoted to something, you can raise money to support it.

Your greatest weakness is lack of self-focus. Here is your rule of thumb: when concentrating on a cause, you might not take care of yourself. It takes a lot of energy to serve. When you're overinvested in a cause, you might be underinvested in your own plights, feelings, or sorrows. Ensure that you're taking care of yourself and watch for these other pitfalls:

- Rigidity. You can get so invested in causes, or prescribe so tightly to ideals, that you become inflexible.

- Judgment. You may feel that everyone should be as dedicated as you are. When they're not? You judge them. Remember: everyone has a different purpose.

- Overly ideological. You may glorify an ideal or organization. If you lack facts, you could waste your time supporting something that doesn't deserve your energy.

- Loss of purpose. When focused on your personal healing, you might not feel quite connected to your higher calling. Yet you must heal internally to fulfill your destiny.

- You're always right. You're not. But you may think you are. Be sure to listen to all opinions before shutting people down.

- Narrow focus. That special cause. It's your thing! Well, there are other things happening in the world, even in your own. Like the need to grocery shop and nurture yourself.

Achieving a harmonious weight. Chances are you won't even know that you're carrying too much weight or don't weigh enough. That's how tuned out you can be. And, as a Harmonizer, you can experience dissonance which can be uncomfortable and lead to paralysis in making choices, food included. Let's face it, it's not pleasant to try to hold two conflicting beliefs at the same time. Waffling back and forth can lead to mediocrity or inaction. So be sure to prioritize your beliefs and create emotional harmony within yourself.

Don't set a weight goal. It's not about pounds or kilograms. It's about how you *feel*. Do you have as much energy in the late afternoon as you do in the morning? Can you sit back and relax when you focus on yourself (which we're insisting you do). If you do perceive yourself as currently under- or overweight, take a trip into Thinker-Land. Yup. Do the Thinker process. Read chapter 6 on the Thinker type to get familiar with the process. Here's a hint: eat several small meals a day with a combo of carbs, proteins, and fats. You'll get to your right set point quickly.

Your chakra organ (in this case muscle) is your diaphragm; you should make all *your food choices with this muscle in mind.* Take a deep breath. You're exercising the strong muscle right below your lungs: your diaphragm. The diaphragm ensures you can inhale oxygen and expel carbon dioxide. In general, your lungs and respiratory system play a key role in creating and maintaining health.

The diaphragm is so important that it's actually the only organ found in all mammals. Without it, animals (like us) would die. Not only is it essential for breathing, but for talking, singing, speaking, and eating. What part of our body *doesn't* require oxygenation?

There are several energetic factors that can support or detract from the functioning of the diaphragm. Your ninth chakra is the point-place for your soul's purpose, which is the reason you are here. How are you serving the greater good? Your breath enables you to cheerlead for your cause. If your breathing is harmonious, you will be too. You'll create coherence in your environment while bringing more light to the planet.

If you're stuck in a critical, judgmental, or victimized place, your body gets tense. In particular, you stop taking full, diaphragmatic

---

CASE STUDY: LASHONDA

LaShonda was run down. Beyond run down. Her husband and children repeatedly pleaded with her to stop all her volunteer activities, which she performed in addition to her day job with a nonprofit.

She admitted that she kept herself going with caffeine and sweets, and kept sleep down to a minimum because otherwise she just felt "hung over." But between her various causes and passions, there was no time for herself or her family.

LaShonda was a classic, overenthusiastic Harmonizer. While she supported ideals that were making the world a better place, this came at great cost to her and her loved ones. The most immediate question was, "What are you running from?"

breaths. If you relate too much to the underdog, you won't fill yourself up. Your heart and lungs will suffer.

FOOD AND SUPPLEMENT PROGRAM FOR THE HARMONIZER

Here are your quick tips for healthy eating.

Quick Tips and Tricks for the Harmonizer

What keeps you in flow as a Harmonizer? Here are some foodstuff tips:

1. Follow a diet based on fruits, vegetables, complex carbohydrates, fish, and lean meats. Eating a balanced diet helps the diaphragm and lungs perform optimally.
2. Assess for food allergies and sensitivities. See a physician, allergist, nutritionist, or naturopath if you need to.

She didn't like that question, but agreed to dig into it, as she was ready to take her health and well-being seriously. After a few weeks, it finally welled up. Her tears flowed. She had been abused by a neighbor as a child. Her parents, both busy with their lives, never noticed her change in attitude or behavior. But almost immediately, she became a vegan—to spare the animals—and started volunteering for various charitable school activities.

Overzealousness is typically an indicator of emotional challenges, but LaShonda's behavior was so extreme, it seemed obvious. After discovering what she had been running from for so many years, LaShonda entered therapy and was more willing to slow down. She immediately adopted a few of the Thinker chakra-type approaches and created a food and exercise schedule for

3. In general, stay away from (or limit) foods that cause gas or a distended stomach. That extra gas puts pressure on your diaphragm and lungs and makes breathing more difficult. We'll point out the most common bloaters in this chapter.

4. Go organic and hormone-, pesticide-, nitrate-, and antibiotic-free, as well as free-range and wild-caught.

5. Eat slowly, sitting up to give your lungs and diaphragm room to expand. After all, eating requires you to chew and breathe at the same time. Eat too quickly and your too-full stomach will press into your diaphragm, creating heartburn, spasms, or hiccups.

6. Eat frequent, smaller meals throughout the day. This can help prevent bloating and heartburn.

7. Don't overeat. Stuffing yourself to discomfort can inflate the stomach. On come the hiccups!

8. Eat spicy and cold foods in moderation. They can irritate or stimulate your phrenic and vagus nerves, which can cause the diaphragm to contract. (Yikes! Hiccups again.)

---

herself. She also shifted her vegan diet, which wasn't giving her enough protein, to vegetarian, allowing herself eggs and other dairy items.

After eating a diet that was less aimed at a cause and more at meeting her nutritional needs, she found herself ready to quit a few of her volunteer activities and reduced her day job to part time. She then joined a running group that was dedicated to fundraising for a cause near and dear. Her daughter, a teenager, participated with her, and her husband and son would meet them at competitions, after which they'd enjoy a family dinner.

On the spiritual level, LaShonda expanded beyond being a "do-gooder." She began connecting with her inner self. Using various yoga breathing techniques, she connected with the suggestion of

9. Limit your salt intake. Too much sodium causes water retention and makes it harder to breathe.

10. Stay hydrated. Drinking lots of water keeps the mucosal lining in the lungs nice and thin. Thick mucus will slow down your respiration.

11. Don't drink fluids with your meals. Try to wait for at least an hour after a meal before you drink water or any other beverage. This prevents you from feeling overly full and gives your diaphragm room to move freely.

12. Load up on the antioxidants. Your best friends? Unsweetened dark chocolate, berries, beets, and pecans.

13. Oxygenate your blood. Do deep breathing exercises and take supplements like chlorophyll, vitamins A, B_9, B_{12}, and C. (More supplement advice later.)

14. Don't eat right before lying down. Try not to nap or sleep (or lie on the couch) for at least three hours after eating. If you're too full when prone, your diaphragm can't function well, and you might end up with heartburn or hiccups.

15. Have no clue about how to create a structured eating plan? Look at the Thinker chapter and follow the basic breadcrumbs. Eat several small meals a day with perfectly balanced portions of carbs, proteins, and fats. As we shared in chapter 3, the Thinker and Harmonizer types are closely related. Many out-of-the-box Harmonizers might do well following the protocol of a Thinker.

---

accessing a personal healing symbol. When visualizing it, she would instantly feel calmer. The LaShonda who emerged from the chakra program was not only happier, but much more harmonized, with herself and with her family.

Food Categories

Let's get into all the foods you should focus on for your optimal health.

Proteins: Go for proteins that are lean and free of chemicals and toxins. Select those rich in omega-3s, which decrease inflammation. Fall in love with salmon, tuna, sardines, cod, sea bass, halibut, and perch. If you're a meat eater, aim for lean proteins like chicken and turkey. Are you a red meat connoisseur? Aim for organic, grass-fed, best-of-the-best options. Then, eat sparingly. Completely avoid cold cuts and processed meats, since the nitrates interfere with the blood's oxygen levels.

Nuts and seeds also provide protein. Eat up walnuts and hempseed, as well as unsalted, organic nut butters.

If you want to get your protein in as a snack, try this spicy nut recipe, loaded with fiber and zinc.

SPICY NUTS

Preheat the oven to 325° F and line a cookie sheet with parchment. Next, mix up a bunch of spices in a bowl big enough to hold a few cups of nuts. Select from ¼ teaspoon cumin, paprika, sea salt, ground cinnamon, ginger, turmeric, cayenne pepper, and black pepper. Are you sort of Italian, at least in nature? Consider oregano, basil, or sage too. Dana's favorite spice mix is rosemary, basil, ginger, cinnamon, and sea salt. To the spices, add 2 tablespoons of olive, avocado, ghee, or coconut oil and stir. Now toss in two cups of walnuts, Brazil nuts, almonds, cashews, pecans, or pistachio nuts—or mix and match! Make sure the nuts get evenly coated and then bake for 15 minutes or so, stirring once or twice. Cool. Package them up and take them wherever you go.

Fats: Your diaphragm and respiratory system require good fats. Olive and avocado oils and healthy nut oils are your friends. Then there are the omega-3 fatty acids found in fatty fish. Want a cooking oil? Choose the monounsaturated fats, like canola and peanut.

Polyunsaturated fats can lower LDL cholesterol and support respiratory health. Keep walnut, sunflower, and flaxseed oils in your pantry. Walnuts, chia seeds, flaxseeds, and sunflower seeds are also good options, providing protein and fats.

Avoid fatty meat fats and trans fats, like partially and fully hydrogenated oils.

Carbohydrates: Your body will harmonize with grains like brown rice and whole pastas. If you eat cereal, consider selecting the fortified brands. Beans and lentils are good in moderation, but if they bloat your stomach, avoid them. (Or give your stomach a couple of days to settle down.) If you overeat carbs, your digestive system will create lots of carbon dioxide, resulting in distension. Consider spreading your carbs throughout the day, and eat them in moderation. Want a trick? Eat protein-based carbs as snacks. Buckwheat is a complete protein. Quinoa is too, and you don't need much to feel full. Make a batch in the morning and heat up a small bowl during the day. Toss in parmesan cheese or nondairy nutritional yeast, salt, and pepper. Or go sweet and throw in a little coconut oil, stevia, and your favorite berries.

Vegetables and Fruits: Think antioxidants and load up on these richly resourced fruits and veggies. Chomp on—or cook—bell peppers, asparagus, tomatoes, and artichokes. Non-starchy veggies are best paired with a carb, limiting the resulting carbon dioxide bloat. Good options? These include leeks, okra, celery, and snow peas. Then go for apples, cherries, plums, pineapple, grapes, peaches, and all berries.

Because your respiratory system is hindered if your stomach distends, be wary of bloating foods. So limit your cruciferous veggies, including broccoli, brussels sprouts, turnips, bok choy, kale, spinach, cauliflower, and cabbage. If you are going to eat them, do so in moderation, and cook them first.

Sometimes a veggie can be the basis for an entire meal. Try our fave recipe below: cheesy roasted asparagus. If you don't do dairy, you can substitute cashew cheese or nutritional yeast. Don't like asparagus? Substitute green beans, broccoli, or a mix of your favorite vegetables.

CHEESY ASPARAGUS (OR SOME OTHER VEGGIE)

Preheat the oven to 400° F. Spread about a pound and a half or two of trimmed asparagus on a baking sheet. Then mix two tablespoons of olive or avocado oil, 4 ounces of mascarpone cheese (or a cheese substitute; we like cashew cheese), 1 teaspoon of salt, ¼ teaspoon of black pepper, and ¼ teaspoon of garlic powder. (If you like garlic, consider adding more garlic powder or adding pressed garlic to the mix.) Then add a dash of cinnamon or turmeric. Stir this mixture for about 30 seconds and pour over your asparagus or other veggie. Sprinkle with the cheese of your choice (or nutritional yeast or a vegan substitute), and bake for about 30 minutes.

Want to boost your diaphragm and lungs with a delicious drink? Try this detox smoothie for healthy yumminess.

BREATH OF FRESH AIR DETOX SMOOTHIE

Add to a blender:

½ cup radish leaves
½ cup spinach leaves
¼ cup diced beets
1 cup liquid of choice (water, coconut milk, or apple juice, whichever is tastiest)
Squeezed juice of 1 lime or lemon

Select and add four of your favorites from among the following fruit ingredients:

1 frozen banana
½ cup frozen mango
½ cup frozen pineapple
½ cup frozen acai
½ cup frozen grapes
½ cup frozen raspberries
½ cup frozen blueberries

Blend until smooth and enjoy this tasty detox.

Dairy: Dairy in moderation is okay—except if you're allergic or sensitive, of course. Dairy contributes to mucous production, so go easy on it. Perhaps you should choose Greek yogurt with no sugar? You can also swap cow milk for a nut milk substitute, like almond or coconut. Oat milk is another possibility, but oats are a grain, so if you're gluten intolerant, be wary. If you don't react to them, eggs are great. Eat both the yolk and the white, as they each contain healthy nourishment.

We know that some of you can't drink dairy, not without lots of problems. So guess what? We're going to share an "ice cream" recipe that really isn't. You'll see what we mean.

PEANUT BUTTER BANANA ICE CREAM, MINUS THE CREAM

Freeze two medium-sized bananas, peeled. Break them in half and add them to a blender, along with ¼ cup of organic peanut butter. Heck, you can also use almond or cashew butter. Like sweetness? Add a little stevia. Want a boost? Dump in some cacao powder. Blend until smooth. Want to turn this into a smoothie? Add coconut or almond milk and blend again. Garnish with roasted, sliced almonds or shredded coconut.

Liquids: Since it's important that you stay hydrated, water and coconut water will be your besties. We recommend alkaline water, which will help to balance your pH levels. Green tea has been shown to decrease inflammation in the lungs, so bottoms up. But coffee isn't a *total* no-no. As a bronchial dilator, it can help open passageways in the lungs, albeit short term. Then again, caffeine is dehydrating, so moderation is key.

Supplements and Spices: We've mentioned salt in the tips for your type. In general, minimize the table salt, but eat foods with iodized sodium. Your diaphragm will thank you, as it needs sodium, magnesium, selenium, and zinc to function well. You can also get these minerals through food, but ask your doctor if a mineral supplement might help. In fact, eating two Brazil nuts per day will give you all your required selenium.

Vitamins A, C, and E are all-important for respiratory health. Vitamin D_3 bolsters diaphragmatic strength and can be gained through fortified cereals or eggs. Talk to your health care practitioner to see if you need a supplement. Consider adding in N-acetyl cysteine (NAC). It supports your immune system while thinning mucus.

Then, take care of your blood. Check your iron levels and supplement if needed. You may also think about adding a chlorophyll supplement to help oxygenate. Vitamin B_3 aids in blood vessel function, so make sure you're getting enough.

Spices? Load up on the ginger, cinnamon, and turmeric, and pretty much all heart-healthy spices. Garlic, onions, and chili peppers are good in moderation too.

The Nopes

We've shared a few already, but we're putting everything in one place, just so you can't say we didn't tell you.

- The whites. We mean breads, pastas, rice, and sugar. And no sneaky or artificial sugars either.

- Sulfites. They can irritate the respiratory system. They are found in wine, beer, shrimp, potato chips, and dried fruits.

- Any food that bloats you.

- Fried foods. Here comes the bloat again. Also, overindulgence in fried foods can cause weight gain, which puts pressure on the lungs and diaphragm.

- Uncooked cruciferous vegetables. These can be hard to break down, and they cause gas and digestive discomfort. If you do indulge, cook them down. Otherwise, opt for carrots, squash, zucchini, romaine, or arugula.

- Carbonated drinks. You'll end up ingesting the carbon dioxide gas, which in large amounts can get all jammed in your digestive system.

- Beer. Darn that carbonation. Cut it out or be careful.

REAL-LIFE EATING TIPS

How will your food prep and practices support you? Here are a few tips.

Food Prep

Come on. You get so busy helping your causes that you don't have time to prep for the week. Right? Wrong. Motivate yourself to pre-cook, chop, and freeze by cooking an extra meal to deliver to a friend or stranger in need. Plan more than one extra meal to deliver to your local shelter if you're feeling extra energized.

Want to skyrocket your enjoyment of a meal? When serving others, have everyone at the table share how they are making the world a better place. Witness others' causes and you won't feel so alone. Dining solo? Say a prayer or wish over your food and ripple out that good energy to all sentient beings.

Grocery Shopping

You've got to feel good about how your food is grown, or you won't shop—and then, you can't eat. Buy local. Search out organic farmers, farmer's markets, or grocery stores that donate their ugly produce to a community center for the homeless. You'll enjoy shopping when you know your ingredients are supporting a better world.

Dining Out

Because you're all about harmony, you'll digest best if you go to low-key, clean-atmosphere restaurants. A restaurant that is too loud—or with an overly robust menu—will stress you out. Check out the vibe before making the reservation. Want to *really* enjoy your food? Make sure the restaurant or food items align with your belief system. Does the restaurant do free-range food, have good hiring programs, or do community outreach? If so, you'll fit right in.

BONUS MATERIAL—BEYOND FOOD

It's not just about food. There are other activities that can support your physical and mental health. Take a look.

Exercise and Movement

Movement will be far more enjoyable when it supports a cause you can get behind. Support a recently opened yoga studio in your neighborhood, join a gym that provides community mentoring, or run a 5k race for diabetes. When there's good as a result of movement, you're more apt to find joy in it.

Yoga will assure flow and harmony, your two "things." A slower-flow yoga will enhance your fluidity and cue breathing. But make sure you get your aerobics in. You need to oxygenate.

If you're feeling uninspired, try an unusual activity—like stand-up paddleboarding or kitesurfing. Get that breath flowing!

Mindfulness and Spiritual Practices

You'll experience personal harmony by activating your intuitive gifts. With practice, you can apply your spiritual gifts to help heal the world—and yourself. We suggest you walk through the following exercises, in the presented order.

EXERCISE: ACTIVATING YOUR UNIQUE HEALING SYMBOL

We want you to discover your healing symbol, an icon that vibrates at your personal frequency. We all have a unique frequency that describes our true selves. By finding and applying this healing symbol, you can be in perfect harmony with yourself and achieve your life purpose. In short, it carries your restorative essence.

1. Breathe deeply and connect with your inner self, as well as your Higher Power.
2. Ask to psychically perceive your personal healing symbol, the representation of your true self. You might intuitively see, sense, feel, or smell it, or even hear its humming.
3. Reflect on this symbol for a few minutes.
4. Create a quick doodle or visual representation of your symbol, or find some other way to be able to remember it at all times.
5. Give gratitude. Thank your Higher Power for this insight and promise to think about or visualize this symbol whenever you are out of alignment and want to reconnect.

EXERCISE: SYMBOLOGY AND FOOD CHOICES

Want to use your gift of symbology to know what food choices to make? You've already obtained your symbol, so the rest is easy. While making a food-related decision, from creating a grocery list to picking a menu item, simply pause for a few moments. Breathe deeply, link with your intuitive self, and connect to your personal healing symbol. Now, sense whether the object of your desire aligns with the symbol. Does it seem that the symbol supports or can encompass the food or beverage item? Does the symbol intuitively glow (that's a yes) or turn dark (that's a no) when you think of selecting a particular menu item? As you work with this activity, you'll soon be able to use this symbol for all foodstuff choices, and even healthy activity choices. Given enough practice, this exercise can aid you in all life decisions.

Sleep and Relaxation

Sleep can elude you when worldly stressors are overwhelming. You have a caring heart, and you can catapult into anxiety. The aroused state can make it really hard to relax or sleep. What's a solution?

Close your eyes and visualize the world you want to live in. This might be your immediate surroundings, the community, or even the global environment. Let yourself feel this world, hear the lovely sounds, smell the fresh and natural aromas. When you are calmed, it will be far easier to fall asleep or return to your everyday life.

Stress-busting and Prevention

Your biggest stressor is the trigger that happens when you can't fix something. And you can't fix everything. So when you're stressed, create a list of the good and meaningful things you *have* done. Revisit this list when you feel down or like you've failed.

Then learn how to perform diaphragmatic breathing. You can follow along to pranayama videos or simply rest a hand on your abdomen and breathe into and out of it. Your nervous system will thank you.

Self-Care Rituals and Needs

You were born to "be the change." But you also need to be yourself. Learn how to focus on yourself and your immediate environment.

Do you like art? Go ahead and decorate your space. Sure, you can purchase art and luxury items that reinforce a benefit, but let yourself choose from your inner, artistic Harmonizer too.

We can't say it enough: you need to breathe. We don't care how you do it, but you might want to sit in a salt studio and breathe in that salty air to clear your lungs. Better yet, get yourself to the beach and take in the negative ions. Can't take a trip? A rushing fountain will work.

SELF-ASSESSMENT QUESTIONS

In order to build your chakra map in part III, you'll want to pick and choose from the concepts and tips provided in this chapter. Spend some time focusing on these questions, and take notes if you can.

1. What's one personal trait that you wish to fully embrace and build on?
2. What's a weakness that you now know to be watchful for?
3. Which foods from the recommended list are your favorites, and should be included in your plan?
4. Which foods from the Nopes list do you need to take out of your current diet?
5. What are some possible substitutions for the Nope foods?
6. What do you fear could be the trip-up point, or downfall, of your new plan? Is there a professional or someone you know who could help you with that?
7. Take stock of your current pantry and food items. Are there any items you should toss out so as not to be tempted?
8. What recommended supplements do you already use, or want to start using, to support your health?
9. Which of the quick tips and real-life tips do you want to use?
10. What grocery shopping and dining habits can you change to help you follow your new plan?

And a few extra questions:

1. What two forms of exercise mentioned for your type appeal to you?
2. What one mindfulness or relaxation technique can you implement when stressed?
3. How about sleep? Is there a way you can improve it? Can you plan better to dedicate more time to nodding off?
4. Select a self-care ritual you know you'll do.
5. Is there another chakra that you would like to strengthen within yourself? If so, what foods or activities can you implement from that specific type to help bolster that chakra within you?

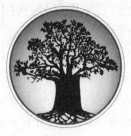

13

NATURALIST

Purpose: Naturalism
You live for nature and love being outside. For you, good health is about respecting and being at one with the Earth. You'll also learn that your tenth chakra links you to the ancestors—your own and those of the cosmos.

Chakra Location: Under the Feet
This chakra is rooted in the ground about a foot and a half beneath your feet. Its endocrine gland is the bones, specifically the bone marrow. Through the marrow, you are constantly in connection with your ancestral genes and your epigenetic process, the shifts in the chemical soup around the genes that toggle them off and on in reaction to what is occurring in your internal or external environment.

Color: Brown
Brown reflects the stability of connecting to the Earth and grounding into your human form.

Chakra Affirmation:
My body is my expression of the Divine.

NATURALIST PERSONALITY TRAITS

Do you roll into work dreaming about your next escape to the outdoors? Are you constantly planning hikes and camping trips and plotting out your cross-country national parks road trip? Or perhaps you spend your hours out in your organic garden, ensuring that your yard is safe for all the bunnies and deer that may call it home. You commune with the earth and love to explore it—for its beauty, its healing vibrations, and the various natural, clean resources it produces.

The call to commune with the environment is beautiful. Ready to learn more?

> **WORDS TO DESCRIBE YOUR NATURALIST SELF:**
> Outdoorsy. Granola. Hippie. Earthy.
> Environmentalist. Green. Hiker. Camper.

Your main intuitive gift is natural empathy. You have the capacity to sense the vibrational qualities of your environment. You can feel when the land is solid, when the trees are happy, and when the flowers need water. But you might also be affected by the movement of the stars and moon above you, the order of the planets, or barometric pressure. The main questions are these: Which of the many beings and places in Nature draw you? What do you want to align with? Do you want to perform animal communication? Cultivate herbal wisdom? Conduct feng shui? It's up to you!

Your major motivator is to experience nature. Your motto? "Get outside!" You love all activities outdoors, whether they involve lying in a hammock, hiking, birdwatching, or stargazing. If you have a dedicated cause, it most likely involves keeping the world in its natural state. Who doesn't want to abolish the plastics in the oceans or for all chickens to be raised free-range? The difference is that you will *act* on your value system.

Your hidden fear is of society's mandates. You have an innate desire to live a life connected to self and to nature. However, your deep, dark fear is that worldly expectations, "should-dos," and responsibilities will keep you from living your heart's desire. The irony? Because of this fear, you tend to shut down and not live your heart's desire anyway. Know that you can be intimately connected to yourself, the environment, and others.

Your greatest strength is your connection to nature. Nature can communicate with and support you in every area of your life. Call upon the many strengths this bond provides you.

- Respect for the Earth. You are keyed in to recycling, composting, and caring for the plant and animal kingdoms.

- Natural healing. It's been said that anything needed for healing is already alive on this good green Earth. Find your specialty area and participate in those protocols.

- Cyclicity. Among all of the chakra types, your body functions most closely to nature's cycles. You can rise at dawn and fall asleep just after dusk. You'll eat healthiest if you select foods grown seasonally and adjust to the ever-changing movement of the moon. Speaking of "cycles," be sure to read the Tree of Life story in this chapter.

- Cosmic woo-woo. How often do you stargaze? What grand messages are being sent from the beings of the stars, or the helpers in the cosmos? Psychically, you can sense these amazing sources of information. Woo-woo maybe, but very cool.

THE TREE OF LIFE: YOUR STORY

There once was a tree that grew strong and proud. It loved to please and provide.

Every spring, the tree showed signs of vibrant life and turned green. Passersby smiled, as eager to support their own rebirth as the tree's renewal. They watered it and sprinkled fertilizer around it. The tree felt good being tended.

When summer came, the tree filled out and provided shade. Oh, it got so hot out! People and their companions walked by, then stopped for a while under the branches. Refreshed, they thanked the tree for its beauty and comfort, even while watering it.

Fall arrived, and the tree offered its sweet fruit. Is it possible that a tree can smile? Maybe, the passersby agreed as they gathered the harvest with glee. "Thank you," they cried, the sweet juices dripping down their chins as they skipped away.

Then, in preparation for the cold weather, the tree began to drop leaves. The people picked them up, using them as mulch or burning them as effigies being offered to the sun. Then the people disappeared. They huddled in their homes and hardly ever thought about the tree.

In its bare, skeletal state, the tree sometimes wondered if it was still loved. After all, the people had disappeared. Even the squirrels stopped leaping about. It had nothing to offer. But then, as always, the tree remembered: it held love in its deep roots, and that love could always be pulled from the depths of the earth. Vulnerable but self-fulfilled, the tree pulled up what it needed, preparing to bloom again come spring.

The tree learned the same lesson every year: to trust the past, accept the present, and know that the sun would shine again.

Your greatest weakness is the tendency to live out your ancestors' issues. In a way, your ancestors are alive within you. Their memories, going back at least fourteen generations, exist chemically inside your genetic material. When triggered, this process of epigenesis can turn your genetic predispositions on and off, causing everything from food cravings to mental or physical illnesses. In addition to watching out for issues that belong to previous generations, watch out for the following:

- Being emotionally closed. You are very rooted. This means you might avoid your personal feelings. When this happens, you might shut down your heart.

- Avoidance of "hard things." When you determine that an action is challenging, or a choice overwhelming, you might avoid taking action or making a choice. That will keep you from experiencing a learning opportunity.

- Escapism. Due to the two aforementioned issues, you may use nature or the outdoors as a way to escape rather than live in your reality.

- Non-development. Since this chakra is hooked into your ancestry, you may accept all inherited family traditions, beliefs, and values, even if they don't match your natural essence.

- Addictions. You may be at risk for addiction to earthly substances that alter emotions and energy; for example, caffeine, sugar, plants that shift your reality, marijuana, tobacco, and alcohol. It's tempting to use these substances instead of working through your feelings.

Achieving a harmonious weight. Balancing at the correct set point, in terms of pounds or kilograms, can be challenging, mainly because you don't always know who you're eating for. Does a particular craving come from you—or from a grandparent whose likes and dislikes are carried in your genetics?

Emotionally, the energy of denial can create imbalances in your weight. Overweight? What feelings are you denying inside yourself?

What are you refraining from speaking out loud? Avoiding in your reality? Underweight? What are you trying to escape or avoid? Utilize your healers for help with this: energy workers, counselors, therapists, and more.

Once you've worked through your emotions, it may be beneficial to check out your ancestral diets. Sometimes the body actually does perform better if we eat like our ancestors did. Some Naturalists also take tips from their blood types. In general, O blood types require animal foods. Type As have a more acidic blood, so they need to alkalize more frequently. If your ethnic background is diverse, use our tips to construct your food plan, or figure out which ancestral strain you most relate to and make sure to add their specific foods.

Your chakra endocrine organs are your bones and bone marrow; you should make all ***your food choices with these in mind.***

Your bones are the framework for your physical self, and metaphysically represent the structure upon which all aspects of your life are built. We don't often think about it, but your skeleton is connec-

CASE STUDY: CHANDA

Chanda was happiest when she was outdoors. The proud owner of three cats and two dogs, she had reason to be outside often. Not only did she frequently walk the dogs, but she had built an outdoor play yard for her kitties too.

When Chanda was home, she had no problem controlling her food choices. She ate organic and hormone-free just about everything, often cooking special meals for her pets as well as herself and her partner. The workplace, however, was her downfall.

Chanda was a veterinarian, and when she thought about it she realized that it was the perfect profession for a tenth chakra Naturalist who loved animals. Except . . . as a tenth chakra Naturalist,

tive tissue. It also produces hormones, which means it's an endocrine gland.

There are three main types of cells that make up your bones: osteoclasts, osteoblasts, and osteocytes. Osteoclasts demineralize the bones. If you have too many, you can get osteoporosis. If you have too few, you can suffer from osteopetrosis. Osteoblasts secrete collagen and minerals, making new bones. They also release the hormone osteocalcin, which stimulates the pancreas to release insulin. Finally, they formulate osteocytes, which become osteoblasts when intertwined in the new bone matrix.

Your bone marrow is just as busy as the bone cells are. It makes white and red blood cells and is vital to just about every function of the body, including your immune system. In fact, most people believe that when we're stressed, the first hormones that kick in are the adrenal hormones. But nope! Get stressed, and the bone marrow produces osteocalcin, which sets off the stress reaction.

From an energetic point of view, bone marrow holds our ancestors' memories and energies. This means that, as a Naturalist, you want to

---

she took on the pain and fear of nearly all her furry, scaly, and feathery patients, often reaching for quick comfort in the form of chips, candy bars, and fast foods. She also despised the ventilated air at the clinic and would come home exhausted, needing to spend a full two hours outdoors to recover.

Most tenth chakra Naturalists are sympathetic with a natural community, whether it's composed of animals, land masses, or stars. Chanda's body simply couldn't cope with the physical and emotional challenges of her community—her patients. Come to think of it, she realized, her father was a cattle farmer who binge-ate carbs and fatty and sugary foods after taking the cattle to be butchered. She also recalled that he drank more alcohol on those evenings too. That meant her epigenetic lineage tied perfectly into her soul sensitivity.

run genetic tests or check for predispositions, as your genes can trigger issues that are latent in your family system.

FOOD AND SUPPLEMENT PROGRAM FOR THE NATURALIST

Are you ready to find out more about your food needs? Read on.

Quick Tips and Tricks for the Naturalist

1. Your best bone diet? One rich in proteins paired with alkalizing veggies, whole grains, and fresh fruits full of antioxidants.
2. Assess for food allergies and sensitivities. If needed, employ a
   physician, endocrinologist, allergist, nutritionist, or naturopath.
3. Go organic and hormone-, pesticide-, and antibiotic-free, as
   well as free-range and wild-caught.
4. Eat protein rich. Your bones need protein. *Lots* of protein.

Chanda was more than willing to adopt a practical eating program, going so far as to pack a week's worth of alkaline-based
snacks every Sunday. She began ordering lunch from a healthy
Asian restaurant, getting in lots of veggies, low-glycemic carbs,
and calcium-rich soy. The most substantial alteration she made,
however, was to her veterinary practice.

Having learned the nature of her soul, Chanda hired a partner. That additional veterinarian did most of the intakes and sur-
gery. For her part, Chanda took an animal communication class
and obtained a certificate in holistic veterinarian care. She then
added a more functional medicine-type approach to the practice and guaranteed that she had the opportunity to spend a few
minutes with each patient, understanding and helping calm them.

5. You'll be happiest selecting foods in cycle with the Earth. Consider the season as well as the time of day. Eat heavier and heartier in the winter, and lighter in the spring. Follow the light of the day with your meals: breakfast at sunrise, lunch when the sun is highest, and dinner at dusk.

6. Avoid sweeteners. If you do need the occasional sweet satisfaction, stevia is your best bet. You could also try coconut nectar or monk fruit. If you use honey, do so in very small amounts.

7. Make friends with alkaline foods. All that protein must be balanced with alkalizing foods. These include chives, cucumber, dandelion, onions, parsnips, peppers, okra, lettuce, leeks, pumpkin, sweet potato, Swiss chard, and radishes.

8. Like orange juice? It likes you. Opt for the kind that's fortified with calcium and vitamin D.

9. Take your vitamin D too. It's a great immune booster and helps the body absorb calcium. Calcium supports the formation of strong bones. To get your vitamin Ds, consume vitamin-rich foods like egg yolks, fatty fish, cheese, or fortified orange juice or cereals. Consult a physician if you think you'd benefit from adding a vitamin D supplement.

10. Get your vitamin C. Our bodies don't produce vitamin C on their own, so we must consume it in our foods or use supplements. Foods high in vitamin C will be listed in the "Vegetables and Fruit" section later in the chapter.

In the offices where she worked most of the time, she had non-fluorescent lighting installed, and she added an air purifier and UV light in the practice's HVAC unit to assure cleaner air. At first, her patients' people thought the approach was a little weird—until, that is, the pets returned home happier and healthier. Her reputation as a stellar vet grew, as did her veterinary practice. Chanda transformed her life to align with her chakra tendencies, and her happiness soared.

11. Know your genetic pitfalls. Consider testing for your genetic predispositions and eating accordingly. Does diabetes run in your family? Watch your sugars. Is Alzheimer's in the gene pool? Reduce your carbs and up those essential fatty acids. You get the picture.

12. Since you're sensitive to your environment, be in tune with your body. If you have odd physical symptoms, check for environmental reactivities, like biotoxin illness, mold sensitivity, chemical sensitivities, air quality, and more.

Food Categories

Here we go! Let's explore all the food-type decisions you should focus on.

Proteins: Healthy bones need healthy proteins. High levels of protein will increase your bone mineral mass as well as build muscle strength. And muscles support your bones. *If* you get the correct balance of calcium, vitamin C, and vitamin D. To figure out your optimal protein intake, have a doctor test your levels.

Ready for the best news? It doesn't matter whether your protein sources are animal or plant. If you eat meat, you'll do well with beef, lamb, chicken, turkey, duck, and pork. To help balance the acids of the proteins and optimize your bone health, pair your proteins with alkalizing fruits and veggies.

If you're vegan, aim for proteins that have a complete amino acid profile. Hemp is a great option, as are quinoa and buckwheat. Include seeds and nuts like sesame seeds, chia seeds, flaxseeds, walnuts, peanuts, pecans, and more.

The reviews are mixed on soy. If you opt to include soy-based proteins like tofu, tempeh, natto, and edamame, pay attention to your estrogen levels. There are claims that soy boosts estrogen; others insist it has an anti-estrogen effect. Talk to your doctor about your best choice.

There are a few alkalizing proteins to choose from as well. These include millet, quinoa, and buckwheat (mentioned earlier), and almonds, sunflower seeds, chestnuts, and watercress.

Fats: Make sure you get lots of essential fatty acids, such as omega-3s. Go for fatty fish, but supplement if you need to, as the body can't make these. Cook with olive and avocado oils. These are good for your bones and your entire body. But it's best to avoid vegetable oils, like corn, soybean, cottonseed, and sunflower. In fact, it's better to cook with fats that are low in omega-6 fatty acids, such as butter and coconut oil.

Carbohydrates: Avoid refined and simple carbs. Your body won't like the acidic residue left behind, nor the potential inflammation. Packaged carbs also mess with your metabolism and can even contribute to insulin resistance. Instead, select whole grains like brown rice, quinoa, and millet. If you eat bread, choose whole wheat, rye, or barley.

Complex carbs like kidney, black, white, garbanzo, and pinto beans are great for their protein and energy boosts. You can put beans in soups, stews, main dishes, salads, tacos, wraps, and chili. Make them a feature in pot pies or stuffed yams. Why not eat kale nachos every so often? Put kale leaves on a cookie sheet or glass pan, after dowsing with olive oil and a little bit of salt and pepper, and toast them in the oven until crisp. Now you have kale chips. Load with heated beans, tomatoes, guacamole, and a little bit of grated cheese. Not much to feel guilty about there.

Vegetables and Fruits: Alkaline. Alkaline. Alkaline. Your body needs alkalizing veggies to counter your mostly acidic protein consumption. The good news is that most veggies are alkalizing. But there are some sneaky ones that leave an acidic residue in your body. So while you indulge in veggies, avoid corn, winter squash, and olives if you're also eating an acidic protein.

Eat lots of leafy greens. Put your steak on a bed of spinach and eat your chicken with an arugula side salad. If it's challenging to put leafy greens in your daily meals, consider a green drink as part of your daily plan. See our formula in this chapter for a bone-building green smoothie using ingredients you have on hand.

Also, consider eating fruits loaded with vitamin C and antioxidants for the double boost to your bones. These include cherries, black currants, berries, oranges, and apples. Luckily, citrus fruits are alkalizing and often high in vitamin C. For this reason, you have the green light to indulge in grapefruit, pomelo, citron, mandarin, lemons, and limes. Kiwi (which is actually a berry) is a good choice too.

Root veggies will harmonize well with your body, since you're so earth connected. Pile on the turnips, onions, garlic, jicama, rutabagas, Jerusalem artichokes, radishes, and ginger. Anything that grows underground is a winner.

BONE-BUILDING SMOOTHIE FORMULA

A simple green smoothie is a great way to ensure you're getting all the ingredients needed for strong bones in one sitting. It's a smart choice to get you going in the morning or provide a quick meal replacement during the day. This recipe gives you the freedom to create a smoothie suited to your taste buds.

Put the following in a blender:

1 cup of leafy greens
1½ cups of chopped fruit or whole berries
1 cup of the liquid of your choice
1 serving of collagen powder or sugar-free protein powder
1 tablespoon of the sugar-free yogurt of your choice (optional)

Here are ingredient options to maximize your bone health:

Leafy greens: collards, kale, chard, broccoli, turnip greens, dandelion greens, parsley, beet greens, watercress, arugula, and spinach.

Fruits: tangerines, oranges, kiwis, papaya, blackberries, prickly pears, mulberries, bananas, figs, clementines, raspberries, lemons, and limes.

Liquid: alkaline lemon water, fortified milk or milk substitute, orange juice.

For an extra punch, you can always add any of the following: chia seeds, flaxseeds, sunflower seeds or sunflower butter, almonds or almond butter, walnuts or walnut butter, cinnamon, and coconut or MCT oil.

Discover your favorite combination or keep mixing it up. Your bones will thank you!

Dairy: Go for it—unless you're allergic or sensitive, of course. We do suggest testing with a physician for lactose or casein intolerance, as these conditions are genetically inherited and common among Naturalists. If you're cow-dairy sensitive, opt for alternatives like almond, rice, or coconut products, especially the fortified versions.

If you get the green light for cow-dairy products, ensure that you're choosing products from cows that are grass-fed or consume organic hormone- and antibiotic-free feed. You can choose milk with extra vitamin D. Also, select fortified yogurt with no sugar. (You can always add a little honey. Consuming local honey will help you fight off potential environmental allergies.)

Cheese is a great source of protein, vitamin D, and calcium. If you're not doing cow cheese, test how you fare with goat cheese. Goat feta, cheddar, and other soft goat cheeses are readily available. If you eat eggs, be sure to consume both whites and yolks: the whites have protein and the yolks are high in vitamin D and phosphorus, all of which are needed for healthy bones.

Liquids: Choose filtered alkaline water with lemon. Remember: you're always looking for ways to alkalize your body. In addition, lemon juice helps you absorb calcium. Fortified orange juice will also give you more zest, but don't overconsume or you'll get too many sugars.

Fortified almond, coconut, rice, and hemp milks are good additions, as is soy if you can tolerate it. Ensure they're organic and hormone- and sugar-free. These can be consumed on their own, as well as in smoothies or decaffeinated teas and coffees.

The jury is still out on carbonated beverages. Some claim the added phosphoric acid can leach calcium from the bones, but the scientific studies have yet to back this up. If you're doing carbonated waters, don't overdo it. Sodas, however, are a nope if they contain sugar or caffeine. Caffeine leaches calcium from the bones, so avoid it. That includes coffee. If you're a coffee lover, find a decaf version you love. Even better, get some dandelion root tea and steep it for an hour or longer. Reheat and imagine that it's coffee. It has a similar taste.

For extra bone bonuses, drink bone broth and collagen water. We've given you a recipe to make your own bone broth (page 260), which has just about everything your bones need for good health.

Supplements and Spices: By now, you've caught on. You need good amounts of calcium, vitamin D, and vitamin C. It's always best to get your vitamins and minerals from foodstuffs, but if you don't consume animal products, consider a vitamin D supplement. Have your D levels and absorption abilities tested, and talk to your doctor about the form to use (whether liquid, capsule, or tablet).

Folate is necessary for the production of white and red blood cells in the bone marrow. Vitamin B_{12} ensures your body produces healthy red blood cells that are circular and small and can move easily from the bone marrow into the bloodstream. Vitamin K aids in bone metabolism and is found in ghee (clarified butter from grass-fed cows. See recipe on page 163), and leafy greens. Parsley is another option. Typically, you can take in enough vitamin K_1 from foodstuffs, which your body then converts to K_2. However, if you have absorption or digestive issues, your body can't alter K_1, so you may need a vitamin K_2 supplement. If that's the case, talk to your doctor. Quercetin, a plant flavonol, lends great support to the bones and can be found in apples and onions.

Iron is needed for bone and blood health. Just don't take calcium and iron at the same time, as your body may not absorb the iron. Magnesium and potassium consumption increases bone mineral density, and resveratrol, which acts like an antioxidant, is like magic for bone health. Not only does it improve bone mineral density, but it encourages bone formation while reducing the breakdown of tissue and loss of bone minerals. Follow up with your physician to see if any of these mineral supplements might help you.

Gram for gram, thyme has more vitamin C than an orange and is also an antioxidant. Other herbs high in antioxidants include dill, sage, peppermint, basil, and oregano, among others. To add flavor to your meals, go for antioxidant-rich spices like cinnamon, cumin, mustard seed, ginger, paprika, and chili powder.

The Nopes

We've already touched on some of these, but here's a more complete list:

- The whites. No white sugar, white flour, white rice, white potatoes, or fake sugars. It's really best not to cheat on the sugar, but if you do, don't do white. Try organic dark chocolate or grab a few dates.

- Acid-forming sides paired with animal protein. Animal protein is acidic in the body, so if you also eat an acidic veggie or fruit, you'll be imbalanced. Go for fruits and veggies and put down the rice and bread.

- Alcohol and nicotine. Both of these can negatively impact your sero-tonin levels.

- Any nonorganic foods or foods raised with hormones or antibiotics.

- Caffeine. Be wary of caffeine, as it upsets your pH levels and pulls calcium from the bones.

- Corn. It's acidifying for the body. This includes all forms, such as corn oil, corn syrup, corn flour, cornstarch, cornmeal, and dextrose.

- Refined carbohydrates. They mess with your metabolism and can lead to increased body fat, which often correlates with decreased bone density. Just say no.

REAL-LIFE EATING TIPS

How can you merge your natural self with your everyday food world? We have some ideas for you.

Food Prep

You will be happiest prepping food that is organic and naturally sourced. Because you're a Naturalist, we recommend cooking as naturally as possible. How about a firepit? Or a grill? Before cooking and eating, pay homage to your Naturalist self, and say thanks to the plants and animals who gave their lives so that you may nurture yourself.

When possible, set up a table outside or, if you live somewhere with a view, in front of a window.

If you own your home and have the means, take a cue from Balinese architecture and consider adding an outdoor kitchen.

Grocery Shopping

Think local and organic. Wherever you go, become a regular. Farmer's markets and local farms will keep your heart happy and make your body healthy. Other Naturalist sorts will hang out in places like this too.

You'll still need run-of-the-mill groceries for staples. Here's a strategy that can help. Create a mainstay list. Separate it into two sections: the supermarket staple list and a farmer's and local market list. Put both lists on your phone so you always have them handy. You can choose different foods each week, but this way your list is available so you won't forget anything. You'll be less tempted to buy those non-organic, sugar-laden cupcakes. After all, even the organic ones are *still* cupcakes, no matter their ingredients.

Dining Out

When you can, opt for outdoor seating. The fresh air will help you digest better. Better yet, dine among the trees. In Japan, thousands of people participate in forest-bathing because trees give off healthy negative ions. But just being around trees is good enough.

Be careful not to overindulge when you're in that farm-to-table, organic restaurant. You'll want to try everything. Don't.

BONUS MATERIAL—BEYOND FOOD

There's more to life than food. Here are some other ways to strengthen and nourish your chakra type.

Exercise and Movement

Hike, mountain bike, kayak, rock climb, swim, paddleboard on the lake, do yoga in the backyard. You can even run in your neighborhood, ski the slopes, snowboard, or kitesurf. Total bonus: goat yoga on a farm.

Because of your connection to the Earth, you may get tempted to give up exercise when you feel emotionally "heavy." But this is exactly when you need it. The endorphins will rev you up and nudge your brain to produce more serotonin.

Though you'll be tempted to forgo indoor workouts for outdoor enjoyment, work in some regular resistance or weight training at least once or twice weekly. This can help maintain and increase bone density.

Mindfulness and Spiritual Practices

Peace equates with being connected to the Earth and outdoor elements. Use the following exercises to ground and harmonize yourself with the Earth's vibration. Then apply this skill to selecting your best foodstuff options.

EXERCISE: CONNECTING TO YOUR ENVIRONMENT

Nature, and everything in it—the stones, plants, and animals—lend soothing and healing energies. Let's help you harmonize with the vibrations of the natural world around you.

1. Find a quiet space outdoors. Stand comfortably (barefoot if possible) and close your eyes.
2. Take a deep in-breath and let it flow all the way to your feet. Then exhale and allow the upcoming breath to bring all your bodily and psychic toxins upward with it. These will exit through your mouth.
3. Perform the above maneuver several times.
4. Now, for a few minutes, let your inhalations reach deep into the earth. As you exhale, the breath brings earth elements upward into your body.
5. Know that the subtle elements of the earth will fill your body and chakra system, leaving you feeling grounded, refreshed, and light. You are now harmonized with Nature and your inner sage.

EXERCISE: YOUR NATURALIST GIFTS AND FOOD CHOICES

Want to use your Naturalist gifts to know what food choices to make? You've already learned to connect to your environment, so you can do that first for extra help.

While making a food-related decision, pause before you choose and connect to the environment through your feet. While focusing on your feet, you're linking with the vibrations most supportive of your body and being. Let this harmonizing energy rise through your body first, and then concentrate on a food-related decision. Sense if this particular food or activity resonates with that vibration. If it reduces your energy, makes you feel heavier, or lowers the oscillation, it's not good for you. If your vibrating energy rises or feels even higher or lighter, you've received a "yes."

Sleep and Relaxation

Sleep under the stars. Okay, you might not be able to literally do that, but there are neat ceiling stars available that you can hang above your bed. In general, flow with the cycles of the Earth. Rise with the sun, and wind down as the sun dips below the horizon. If you work late with computer screens, invest in blue light–blocking glasses so you can sleep better.

Meditating outdoors at dusk will establish your circadian rhythms for a solid night's snooze. Can't go outside to meditate and calm your mind? Bring the outdoors in. Fill a living space with plants and maybe even a fountain, and relax in this space. You'll drift off better in your bedroom with nature soundtracks or open windows.

In need of a relaxation reset? Make a date outside. You and the sky. You and the ocean. You and the mountains. You and the land.

Stress-busting and Prevention

The best stress prevention for you is regular outdoor time or engagement with animals or the environment. Volunteer once a week at a no-kill animal shelter; better yet, get a pet. There's nothing like a dog; they'll force you to go outside. Admit it—you want to be out there anyway. Again, if you can't care for a pet, do something for animals, even if it's providing financial support for a rescue center.

When you're in the great outdoors, close your eyes and take some deep breaths. Put one hand over your heart to remind yourself it's safe to be open and loving.

Self-Care Rituals and Needs

There are two sides to a coin. The first, we've covered: get outside regularly. But also, do something that involves the natural world, like a hobby. Woodwork, gardening, birdwatching. You get it.

The second recommendation might feel like an indulgence, which is the point. Pamper yourself. Get an updo or a makeover. And try massage, acupuncture, infrared saunas or salt rooms, or some other type of nurturing body care.

SELF-ASSESSMENT QUESTIONS

In order to build your chakra map in part III, you'll want to pick and choose from the concepts and tips provided in this chapter. Spend some time focusing on these questions, and take notes if you can.

1. What's one personal trait that you wish to fully embrace and build on?
2. What's a weakness that you now know to be watchful for?
3. Which foods from the recommended list are your favorites and should be included in your plan?
4. Which foods from the Nopes list do you need to take out of your current diet?
5. What are some possible substitutions for the Nope foods?
6. What do you fear could be the trip-up point, or downfall, of your new plan? Is there a professional or someone you know who could help you with that?
7. Take stock of your current pantry and food items. Are there any items you should toss out so as not to be tempted?
8. What recommended supplements do you already use, or want to start using, to support your health?
9. Which of the quick tips and real-life tips do you want to use?
10. What grocery shopping and dining habits can you change to help you follow your new plan?

And a few extra questions:

1. What are two forms of exercise mentioned for your type that appeal to you?
2. What one mindfulness or relaxation technique can you implement when stressed?
3. How about sleep? Is there a way you can improve it? Can you plan better to dedicate more time to nodding off?
4. Select a self-care ritual you know you'll do.
5. Is there another chakra that you would like to strengthen within yourself? If so, what foods or activities can you implement from that specific type to help bolster that chakra within you?

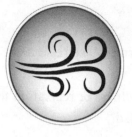

14

COMMANDER

Purpose: To Command
As an innate leader, you can access both natural and supernatural powers. Your foods must support and sustain the courage and stamina needed to make great changes in the world.

Chakra Location: Connective Tissue
How is the connective tissue an organ? Most hormone glands are embedded in the connective tissue. In turn, connective tissue is affected by hormones. Even more importantly, the job of the connective tissue—as well as the muscles that serve as your secondary bodily system—is to hold the entire body together. Isn't that what leadership is all about? You link people and energies to reach an established goal.

Color: Rose
Rose is a combination of red, which represents physical authority, and white, symbolizing spiritual purity. In short, you merge the mundane and the esoteric to catalyze change.

Chakra Affirmation:
I am an instrument of Divine power.

COMMANDER PERSONALITY TRAITS

Mix a super-powered personality with commanding forces and you end up with—*you*. Your physical health is predicated on your ability to make ethical, integrated choices about what you can and cannot see or touch.

Let's delve into your Commander personality.

WORDS TO DESCRIBE YOUR COMMANDER SELF:
Bossy. Leader. Empowered. Integrated. Alchemist. Catalyst. Trailblazer. Forceful. Achiever. In charge.

Your main intuitive gift is force empathy. What in the world is force empathy? Basically, you can summon and direct natural and supernatural energies toward an objective. Need a little wind to dry the sweat on your body? Order it up! Or maybe you'd like to send a *helpful* spell to better someone's day. You have the ability.

In the end, you access and direct forces using your willpower. We'll present an exercise to educate you about these basic forces—there are twelve of them—and show you how to employ their energies, which can alter the world for the better.

Your major motivator is to lead. You are a leader. It doesn't matter whether you're interfacing with ordinary or extraordinary forces or wielding common or uncommon authority. The best leaders are also followers. What better to follow than your own food program?

Your hidden fear is that you will be abusive or do harm with your power. Perhaps you've been on the receiving end of someone abusing their power. Or maybe you've simply seen enough of it in the world around you. Here's the thing: develop your heart, hone your kindness. Then your power will amplify those things. And the world can use way more of that.

Your greatest strength is your commitment to achievement. You aren't the type to sit around while others make things happen. You compel successes.

Under your leadership, any group is bound to reach a high point. Then again, you might be a solo Commander. Being a leader doesn't mean you're always in charge of a community. Writers, painters, healers, and even independently employed accountants can be Commanders. The distinguishing factor is that you point, aim, and move.

A Commander must always be on point for themselves. Do this by drawing on your strengths, which include the following:

- Steadfastness. See that mountain? Whether it's internal or external, you'll climb it. Tenaciously.

- Mastery. How do you want to focus your powers? You are not only good, but great at whatever you undertake.

- Self-assurance. You won't try to do something if you don't think you can.

- Strategic planning. Think of successful generals. They have vision. You can get anywhere if you know where you're going.

- Agility. Does it matter if someone or something gets in the way? Not really. You can jump over a boulder as easily as you can outmaneuver an opponent.

Your greatest weakness is grandiosity. Power-based people sometimes get caught up in their own power. There are lots of pitfalls related to grandiosity. Get familiar so you can avoid them.

- Egoism. It's easy to think you're better than others because you're great at what you do. That can be a mistake.

- Bossiness. You're super at being in charge, but no one likes a know-it-all.

- Negativity. You have an innate ability to uncover the silver lining in the cloud, but you can also get lost in the storm. Be sure to engage with the sunny side of life.

- Overeating. What?! Can't any chakra type overeat? Of course. But you put so much energy out there that it's pretty easy to compensate with food.

- Sensitivities. Being attuned to forces can make you sensitive to them. You can easily take on others' depressive or anxious moods or swing with planetary and climactic shifts. Astute self-awareness will help you differentiate between what applies to you and what to ignore.

Achieving a harmonious weight. You are so busy leading that you don't pay attention to how much or how little food you're eating. For the Commander, food is merely an obstacle to making things happen, a necessary evil that must be addressed. That means you'll either overeat or undereat. Follow our advice and you'll adjust to an optimum weight.

Sometimes a Commander's body holds too many pounds because weight can be subconsciously associated with power and force. And powerlessness is a Commander's worst fear. It can lead to issues with food: overeating to stuff the feeling or undereating because you feel you don't deserve the nourishment or are afraid of your own power. If this is your issue, learn about your intuitive gifts through the exercises found later in this chapter. But know this: you really can direct forces. Do that with your mind and willpower and your body won't have to be weighted down in order to push you (or others) forward.

Own your power and balance it with your loving heart. Overall, work with your intuitive gifts to become comfortable being in charge, and your weight will stabilize.

*Your chakra endocrine gland is your connective tissue; you should make **all** your food choices with this gland in mind.* On the physical level, connective tissue supports and surrounds organs and other body parts. Collagen and elastin are two main ingredients of fatty tissue, cartilage, and bones. They help bind, support, protect, insulate, store fuel, and move substances throughout the body.

Connective tissue doesn't make hormones itself, but most of the endocrine glands are found embedded in connective tissue. Although endocrine glands secrete hormones into the bloodstream, many of these hormones must first pass through connective tissue.

One particular type of connective tissue, the fascia, is extraordinarily important. Fascia is a band of connective tissue, primarily made of collagen, that lies beneath the skin. It attaches, separates, and stabilizes muscles and other internal organs. Bodyworkers and other types of healers have observed that clients' memories are often invoked when they are working on the fascia. What does this memory-filing capability mean for you, the Commander? You have a capacity for digging into your own connective tissue to intuitively connect with age-old leadership and magical skills.

CASE STUDY: ALEJANDRO

Alejandro loved his life—for the most part. He ran a successful service company, was the proud father of four children, and made enough money so that his husband could stay home and tend to the busy lives of the kids. But for all his trying, he couldn't eat a healthy diet. Nor did he force himself to exercise, except on the weekends. And then, more often than not, his insane, warrior-like, once-a-week workout left him aching and then eating endless amounts of pasta for comfort and energy.

Alejandro was willing to change, but had no idea how to do it.

He warmed to the idea of being a Commander. Smiling, he admitted that people had always followed his lead, even in school. "If there was a committee, I usually ran it," he declared. In his profession, his clear sense of vision and action had attracted more customers and dependable employees than most in his line of business. He deserved to be proud. However, he was so busy meeting his work targets and caring for family that he didn't set personal health goals for himself.

Alejandro was happy to create a health initiative for himself, though he had no idea how he was going to keep it up. "There are always emergencies," he complained. "How can I guarantee that I'll go to the gym four times a week?"

He couldn't. Alone, that is. So, at our suggestion, he decided to engage in agreements with his main work staff, his husband, and his kids. At work, he and his fellow team leaders established new protocols for the workplace that included the availability of healthy food and time off for meditation and exercise. At home, he and his husband established similar agreements. "Whole health, whole family" became their motto. Alejandro and his husband started grocery shopping together and preparing healthy meals and snacks twice a week. During dinnertime each night, they took turns "giving the floor" to a different family member. That person would initiate whatever discussions they wanted to. Alejandro took daily walks with either his husband or one of the kids. He also agreed to coach for one child's soccer team, which required him to run around every so often, not only once a week.

Over time, Alejandro noticed an anomaly in his leadership skills. Sometimes he could decide that something supernatural would happen—and it would. When their garden was dry, he wished that it would rain. It did. Alejandro hasn't yet figured out what he wants to do with this strange ability, but we're sure he will.

FOOD AND SUPPLEMENT PROGRAM
FOR THE COMMANDER

Let's go over the ways you can best nurture and support your Commander self.

Quick Tips and Tricks for the Commander

How can you command a food program? Here are a few ideas:

1. Pretend you're in boot camp. If you approach your food program like it's super serious (and there is a medal at the end), you'll follow it.
2. Don't over-chow. Unless you're burning 10,000 calories a day, you don't need to consume that many.
3. Keep all your endocrine glands happy. As we've said, your connective tissue houses most of your endocrine glands. You can keep them healthy by avoiding the bad stuff like MSG, nitrates, chemicals, and more. If you eat meat or dairy, choose lean and grass-fed, organic, hormone-, pesticide-, and antibiotic-free sources or full-amino acid proteins, and only organic veggies and fruits and the good fats.
4. If you're building muscle, something a Commander loves to do, detoxify every few months. The secret is lots of water. In fact, joint cartilage is about 60 percent water.
5. Assess for food allergies and sensitivities. Talk to a physician, endocrinologist, allergist, nutritionist, or naturopath.
6. Consider saying good-bye to gluten. This protein, found in grains like wheat, rye, and barley, can cause inflammation. Cow milk can also be tough on the digestive system, so be aware of your tolerance for it, or lack thereof.
7. You're a beast. To compensate for all that pushing, whether physical or mental, get plenty of antioxidants and anti-

inflammatory foods. We'll give you lots of ideas, but one deserves to move to the top of the list: bone broth stocks. The gelatin is anti-inflammatory and will provide lots of accessible amino acids.

8. Go for catechins and anthocyanins. What are these? Phytochemicals that stitch collagen fibers together. We'll give you some examples later.

9. Don't "diet." You are a mover and shaker. You will muscle your way through anything and everything. Keep your metabolism stoked by not dieting. Just eat healthy. Muscles actually burn more calories than fat does anyway.

Food Categories

All right! Time to zero in on all the types of foods a Commander should choose.

Proteins: Collagen and elastin, the two main ingredients in connective tissue, are made of protein. So are your muscles. In short, you need lots of proteins, especially those that contain the complete amino acid panel.

If you eat meat, go for grass-fed beef and bison and organic chicken and turkey. Wild-caught salmon delivers anti-inflammatory omega-3 fats. Reach for other fish too, including tuna and scallops; the latter are especially low in fat. Think prawns, also. They have lots of glucosamine, which you need for connective tissue health.

Eggs or tofu, anyone? Yes! Then add in black beans, lentils, and nuts such as almonds, cashews, and walnuts. If you're looking to bulk up, organic peanuts add calories. Healthy choices also include seeds like flax, chia, and hemp. Sesame and pumpkin seeds have lots of zinc, an important mineral for your tissue. Those sesame seeds also deliver copper, a required mineral, as do sunflower seeds.

If you're into beans, add pinto and kidney to your beans list, and also chickpeas. Though edamame isn't an official protein, these immature soybeans pack a protein punch, guaranteeing around 17 grams of protein and 8 grams of fiber per serving. Just saying.

MAKE GOOD BONES WITH BONE BROTH

Bone broth is good for your bones on every level, and it's easy to make.

Save the bones from organic roasted chicken or beef (or buy bones from the butcher), or the shells from shellfish, and put them in a large pot. Throw in a few lemon wedges and add rosemary and thyme, if you like those seasonings. Cover with about 12 cups of water and add about 1 tablespoon of salt and 2 tablespoons of apple cider vinegar. If you want an extra punch, add in some of your favorite alkalizing veggies. Bring the broth to a boil and then reduce to a simmer. Simmer for about twelve hours. Strain and store in the refrigerator for up to three days, or in the freezer for up to a year. You can drink it like a tonic or make a soup with it. Just toss in some vegetables, miso, garlic, onions, and other tasty additions. It's also a great substitute for gravies and sauces.

Fats: We can't say it enough. Omega-3s. Omega-3s. Omega-3s. Your connective tissue and muscles crave omega-3s. And your body doesn't make them on its own. Besides that, your selection of fats can be pretty common sense. Healthy fats provide 70 percent of your body's energy at rest and help maintain testosterone, which builds muscle.

Our advice? Cut out saturated and trans fats, such as vegetable oil fats, and especially hardened margarine. Stoke your endocrine glands and tissues with monounsaturated fats, including olive and peanut oils. Avocado oil is also a good choice.

Carbohydrates: Even though Commanders adore protein, carbs keep you going. They enable you to get more done quicker. For your carbs, select nutritious sources that enable glycogen storage. Glycogen, mainly stored in the liver and muscles, is a form of glucose that provides energy when needed. A short list of healthy options includes yams, sweet potatoes, other root veggies, legumes, winter squash, buckwheat, and quinoa. Buckwheat and quinoa are especially terrific for a Commander, as they are both a full protein and a carb.

Most of the Commanders we know refrain from gluten, which can be very sticky and inflammatory for the system. Test it out for yourself, though. Also, go for whole grains. Buy that brown rice cooker and indulge in vegetable pastas for extra nutrition.

If you're crushing those muscle-building workouts and burning through calories, whip up some post-workout mashed sweet potatoes. Add a little coconut milk, some coconut water to restore your electrolytes, avocado oil, and cinnamon. Top with blueberries and carrot shavings if you desire. This concoction will taste like dessert and restore your glycogen levels. Rice cereal is super easy to digest, and you can dress it up nutritionally with a banana or raisins, maybe even mixing in cottage cheese, if you do dairy.

How about baking a few bran muffins laden with sunflower and chia seeds, but substituting monk fruit or honey for sugar? Heck, add some whey, pea, and hemp protein and you'll be ready for a pre-workout boost or a post-workout recovery. No downtime? Turn to a quinoa-based low- or no-sugar cereal.

Vegetables and Fruits: We're going to start with an oddball recommendation. Okra. Ever tried it? Okra lubricates dry tissue. Dehydrated okra, or okra in a vegetable soup, is fantastic.

Overall, broccoli and cauliflower are great in that they contain sulfates, which combine with chondroitin to form cartilage. Avocados include copper, which your connective tissue requires, and who can resist guacamole? Kale is another healthy option, as are mustard greens and arugula.

Let's look for those anthocyanins. (We're sure you're still trying to pronounce that word, and good luck.) Think purple, blue, and red plants. The list of veggies and fruits containing them include acai, blueberries, eggplant, black currants, blackberries, cranberries, cherries, red or dark grapes, guava, pomegranates, red cabbage, and red onions. Try a Peruvian drink that will give you lots of these powerful disease-fighting flavonoids. In a blender, mix 2 cups of chopped guava and 2 cups of pomegranate seeds. Add a tablespoon of stevia and ½ teaspoon of salt. Blend it up, strain it, and drink away.

Catechins are another type of flavonoid that helps your cellular health. Acai, peaches, apricots, plums, and nectarines are good sources.

You also need a lot of vitamin C. Try papaya, oranges, kiwi, pineapple, and strawberries.

Dairy: Always test your ability to tolerate dairy with your doctor. If dairy is a yes, you're in luck. Eggs are a mainstay. High in cysteine, they are a great source of protein, healthy fats, vitamins, and cholines. Greek yogurt has twice the protein of regular yogurt, and cottage cheese is a super muscle-building snack. Tofu, made from soy milk, also appears on our protein list and is considered a fantastic plant-based protein.

Let's talk milk. If you can tolerate cow milk—and many people can't—it's a great way to increase muscle mass, in combination with weight training. Plus, it's considered good for tissue repair. For some people, raw dairy is the way to go. Kefir is also an option.

Liquids: Drink a lot of water. After all, 70 percent of the body is water, and your connective tissue requires lots of it. Green tea has catechins, which prevent the breakdown of collagen. Kombucha is a terrific add too! This fermented tea can aid with detoxification.

We're not totally against red wine either. The odd glass there and again promises a few catechins, and maybe a little relaxation.

Supplements and Spices: There are lots of smart supplements and spices that will strengthen your connective tissue and muscles. Of course, the best source for your required vitamins and minerals? Real food! However, we understand that sometimes you need a little extra support, so we'll cover a few of the nutrients for which you may want to use supplements.

Put zinc high on the list, as it's required to make cartilage and bone. Vitamin C creates and forms collagen. Glucosamine, most of the B vitamins, vitamin K, magnesium, glutamine, and lipoic acid are underpinnings of connective tissue workings.

Been a weekend warrior and now you're paying for it with sore joints? Say this after us: superoxide dismutase (SOD). It will reduce joint tissue inflammation. You can also reach for spirulina. Vitamin E, too, is a heavy hitter for tissue repair.

The stronger your muscles, the better you'll be able to direct both natural and supernatural forces. Some of the most respected supplements for gaining muscle mass include creatine, protein supplements, the amino acid beta-alanine, branched-chain amino acids (BCAAs), and beta-hydroxy beta-methylbutyrate (HMB). Some would-be athletes like whey protein for a supplement; they also take a lot of fish oils. Better yet, work with a darn good nutritionist or health care professional to learn how to mix and match all these supplements.

Here are some other interesting supplements you may want to look into. Nettle leaf is high in calcium, magnesium, and iron. If you want silica to strengthen your tissue, aim for alfalfa leaf and horsetail. For calcium, try oat straw. Marshmallow root and Solomon's seal lubricate dry tissues, while turmeric, ginger root, and white willow bark are anti-inflammatories. If you have damaged tissue you'd like to heal, go for mullein root and gotu kola.

When you're cooking, slice, dice, and slather on the mustard, garlic, and onions. The sulfates in them combine with chondroitin to create cartilage.

If you're in need of a little fun, organic dark chocolate (with a healthy sweetener like monk fruit or stevia) or cacao fit on your treats list. They have lots of anti-inflammatories and catechins.

The Nopes

You've probably figured out a bunch of your Nopes. We'll underline a few here anyway so you can keep them in mind.

- The whites. No white sugar, white flour, white rice, or white potatoes— except if you're intensely physically training. In that case, consume white rice and potatoes in moderation. But don't cheat with that white sugar—or the fake sugars.

- Fatty foods, like butter, meat, and fried foods. Bad fats interrupt endocrine gland functions.

- Packaged and frozen foods. Honestly, these aren't "actual" foods, so when you can, cook.

- Alcohol. Except for that occasional red wine.

REAL-LIFE EATING TIPS

How do you navigate those real-life food decisions? Here's how!

Food Prep

Put yourself in charge of your food prep, whether for a meal or the week. If you assign yourself the job, you'll do it. Really don't want to? Embrace team action. Put your kids, friends, or partner to work as chefs or sous chefs. Or, if you're able, you can always hire some professional food prep help.

Grocery Shopping

You are a quick-action person. Short of sending someone else to do your shopping, or ordering it online, do your shopping once a week. Make a list, check it twice, and get it done.

You'll feel less frustrated if you don't shop in big crowds. Avoid shopping on Sunday afternoon, at lunchtime, or during pre-dinner hours. Plan a few meals in advance so you know what to buy. Because you'll be loading up for a week, grab perishables from the back of the shelf. Those will last the longest, as they are most recently stocked.

Dining Out

Here's the thing. You can be an annoying dining companion. Do you find yourself trying to order for yourself *and* your company? Do you tell the waiter exactly how to cook the steak? We don't mean temperature, as in medium or medium rare. We mean you're directing the chef as to when to flip the steak on the grill. By the way, if you *must* order for your dining mate, ask for their permission first.

BONUS MATERIAL—BEYOND FOOD

Health is about so much more than food. What other activities can you undertake to maintain Commander standards?

Exercise and Movement

Here is our advice. Undertake exercises that target your connective tissue and also strengthen your muscles. In short, go for the collagen-building workout. How? Perform light sets of low-impact exercises, which can include reverse lunges and calf raises. Get and keep your tendons and ligaments in shape and then add in the muscle-growing lifts.

What else will propel you into Commander shape? Use full-body exercises, and take advantage of your desire to lead and achieve. Join a team and you'll work hard, so as to never let your teammates down. Better yet, spearhead a team and you'll keep yourself healthy as the head of the pack.

Mindfulness and Spiritual Practices

Leaders can't make clear decisions if they're distracted or overly focused, or if they're being reactive instead of proactive or responsive. This is true whether you're in charge of people, animals, plants, or energy entities. That's why we're giving you an exercise that will clear your brain and also show you how to summon and direct subtle forces.

What are these natural and supernatural forces we keep talking about? Whether visible or invisible, these forces are made of natural energies, such as fire, water, and wood.

EXERCISE: GOODBYE, TOXIC BRAIN—HELLO, COMMANDER OF FORCES

This process will help you access power and clear your chattering mind.

1. Stop. Stand still. Then move in place. We know—that's a weird order. But it works for you. While standing, twitch your muscles, shuffle your feet, and wave your hands.
2. Now, create an energy ball. Here's how:
   Hold the palms of your hands in front of you, facing each other, about three inches apart. Close your eyes and visualize the back of your heart opening. Let your intuitive smarts select which of the many subtle energy forces you want to stream through the back side of your heart, down your arms, and into your hands. Your choices are as follows:
   Water: Flow and freedom, cleansing of emotions
   Wood: Optimism and initiative
   Fire: Purification and energy
   Air: Release of negative thoughts and influx of positive truths
   Metal: Protection against evil and transmission of guidance
   Earth: Fortification and repair

Ether: Higher consciousness and spiritual illumination

Star: Energizing of high ideals and goals

Stone: Access to historical and ancient knowledge

Sound: Creation of power—the "oomph" needed to make something happen

Light: Formation of love to support connection

Presence: The sense of a Higher Power

3. Mix the subtle forces. Stream through as many as you like. Allow these incoming energies to blend in between your hands. As they fuse, they create a single force.

4. Program. Create a strong statement that encapsulates what you want to achieve. Then mentally send that intention into the energy ball. To clear the mind, you can use a focus statement, such as "I now clear the debris out of my mind." You can also decide upon something you want to manifest or heal.

5. Move your hands. Gesture in a way that underscores your fierce intent. For instance, you can wave your hands over your head to erase negative thoughts. You can throw the energy ball into the air—and into the world—while thinking about a desire. Remember not to use this with a negative or harmful intention, for yourself or anyone else. It will circle back and cause you problems.

6. Clear your hands and close. When finished, pat your hands together and release the built-up energy before returning to your daily life.

Sleep and Relaxation

Even if you seem to be a Type B personality, your inner workings are all Type A. Type As tend to think their checklist is more important than rest and relaxation, but guess what? Sleep is the foundation for optimal performance. So follow this list to get out of high drive:

• No energy drinks past 3:00 p.m. They will push your adrenals into an obnoxious overdrive, and you'll be too wired to sleep or kick back.

- Turn off the screens by 7:00 p.m.

- Only do perceptual, not conceptual, activities from 7:00 p.m. onward, or when on vacation. Conceptual actions, such as reading and talking, are hard. They make your brain overwork. Perceptual? These include light walking, doing the dishes, and being playful.

- Stop eating two hours before bed. You don't need those digestive juices stirring you up.

Stress-busting and Prevention

We have two simple pieces of advice. You'll want to do each one every day. The first? Be a boss-leader. Force yourself to accomplish a huge goal every day. Not gigantic by someone else's standards, but big by your own. Lift that boulder or command that windstorm. Put away those clean clothes, finish up your taxes, or implement those new guidelines for your business. The second task? *Don't* be the boss. Do something passive. Binge-watch that cool show or go to a movie chosen by a friend.

Self-Care Rituals and Needs

Get a mentor. In fact, we suggest two mentors. The first should be living. Let them connect you to your soft, romantic side. The second can be either living or otherworldly, but for sure, should be a master of spiritual forces. You'll know them when you find them.

SELF-ASSESSMENT QUESTIONS

In order to build your chakra map in part III, you'll want to pick and choose from the concepts and tips provided in this chapter. Spend some time focusing on these questions, and take notes if you can.

1. What's one personal trait that you wish to fully embrace and build on?
2. What's a weakness that you now know to be watchful for?

3. Which foods from the recommended list are your favorites and should be included in your plan?

4. Which foods from the Nopes list do you need to take out of your current diet?

5. What are some possible substitutions for the Nope foods?

6. What do you fear could be the trip-up point, or downfall, of your new plan? Is there a professional or someone you know who could help you with that?

7. Take stock of your current pantry and food items. Are there any items you should toss out so as not to be tempted?

8. What recommended supplements do you already use, or want to start using, to support your health?

9. Which of the quick tips and real-life tips do you want to use?

10. What grocery shopping and dining habits can you change to help you follow your new plan?

And a few extra questions:

1. What are two forms of exercise mentioned for your type that appeal to you?

2. What one mindfulness or relaxation technique can you implement when stressed?

3. How about sleep? Is there a way you can improve it? Can you plan better to dedicate more time to nodding off?

4. Select a self-care ritual you know you'll do.

5. Is there another chakra that you would like to strengthen within yourself? If so, what foods or activities can you implement from that specific type to help bolster that chakra within you?

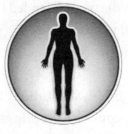

15

TWELFTH CHAKRA

> **Chakra Affirmation:**
> I am Divine.

This chapter is shorter than our other chakra chapters, yet it's equally important. Maybe even more important. You'll understand better after we describe your twelfth chakra and the very special reason you need to access it.

You've always known there is something special about you. A way of being—and doing—that is unique. Perhaps you've never spoken about this inner sense with anyone before, but we want to speak about it with you now.

Your twelfth chakra is home to your most extraordinary intuitive gift, which is unique to you. No one else has the special gift that you do. No one.

Ready to learn more about this chakra, as well as how to understand and activate your exceptional gift? Let's go!

WHAT'S YOUR TWELFTH CHAKRA?

Your twelfth chakra is distinct to you. It is basically made up of your true self's extraordinary subtle energies. Within this chakra lies an intuitive gift unlike anyone else's.

From a subtle perspective, this chakra is found in several places. It is interwoven with your twelfth auric field, which lies at the outer perimeter of your auric field. It connects into your physical body through thirty-two different points. But it is most accessible in the center of your heart chakra.

If perceived as a color, or as a set of colors, this chakra's appearance would be particular to you. Some people see their essence as a single hue, and others as a rainbow splash. Still others regard it as translucent or opaque.

The exclusive gift contained within your twelfth chakra is more than a "nice to know" ability. Learning to activate and use it is vital to achieving your soul's purpose. You can also apply this inner talent to make important foodstuff decisions.

Want an example of an exceptional power? Here is a great one.

Cyndi once worked with a woman over the phone who refused to tell her anything about herself. Intuitively, Cyndi perceived this woman as being a princess who had married a prince in a castle. The woman laughed. Confiding in Cyndi, she said that she actually *was* a princess, although a very minor one. She had also married a real-life prince, albeit not one high on the totem pole. And guess what? They were wed in a castle.

Having struck a chord, Cyndi was next shown this woman's very special aptitude.

"If you write a story for someone," Cyndi shared, "the ending will come true."

The client gasped. "That has happened three times!" she exclaimed.

The client had written a fable for three different people and, sure enough, the stories' conclusions had come to life. A little boy had healed from leukemia. A woman who had been unemployed for two years got her dream job. A man excommunicated from his family was welcomed back with wide-open arms.

There are as many special gifts as there are people. Additional examples include a woman who can sense the exact origin of another's illness, a man who writes such beautiful poetry that everyone who hears it either cries or laughs, and a girl who can create paintings that deliver healing energies.

To Cyndi's knowledge, the storyteller hasn't used her innate gift since that intuitive session. Sometimes we are afraid of what makes us wonderful—we'd rather just keep wonder*ing*. For that reason, we've included a final part II action step for you, in the form of the following exercise. We'll be asking you to commit to using and developing your ability. Sure, we'll help you apply it to your food program. We also want you to consider employing your newfound aptitude in other areas of your life—or any place you perceive it can benefit humanity and the world.

Exercise: Lighting Up Your Very Special Gift

It's time to uncover and apply your unique and divine gift. To do this, follow these instructions:

1. Let yourself get quiet. Take a few deep breaths and settle into the center of your heart chakra. Within this haven of purity, connect with your own vital spirit. This is the self that knows itself as divine.
2. Assess this central core. How do you perceive this essential self? What color or colors pop into your mind? What sensations, feelings, aromas, or other descriptors might help you describe your essential self? Identify as many aspects of this, your essence, as you can.
3. Activate your inner light. It's time to fully initiate your inner essence. In turn, all other facets of your twelfth chakra will awaken, including your special ability. Simply ask your inner,

wise self or Higher Power to fully awaken within your heart core. If you are visual, you will perceive a blaze of your natural, spiritual light. If you are more verbal, you'll hear a sound, tone, or song illuminating your truth. If you are sensory, you'll feel the expansion of your personal energy.

4. Embrace your special gift. Allow your inner sage to reveal this extraordinary ability. What images do you receive to explain how you might express it? Deliver it? Label it? What else do you need to become aware of? Know that you'll receive responses now, and more as time goes on.

5. Gratitude and commitment. Feel grateful for—yourself! For the gifted, rich being of light you are. Then commit to applying your gift in all that you do.

APPLYING YOUR TWELFTH CHAKRA GIFT WHEN MAKING FOOD CHOICES

We can't tell you exactly how to apply your twelfth-chakra ability toward creating the perfect food and lifestyle program for you. That's because you are unique. We can, however, ask you a series of questions that will invite reflection and aid decision-making. Your answers will be integrated in part III on your chakra map.

1. How would you describe your special spiritual gift in a single sentence?
2. How can knowing this ability inform your long-term decisions?
3. How does knowledge of this aptitude help you perceive your main chakra and its foodstuff needs?
4. Which foodstuffs will help you best support the use of your special quality?
5. Which foodstuffs should you abstain from?
6. What lifestyle activities might enhance and contribute to this gift?

7. Is there a way to use this ability when you are making food choices in the moment? When grocery shopping? When dining out? When performing some other food-related activity?

8. Is there anything else you need to know about your special gift that will help you create a food program that is perfect for you and you alone?

This chapter concludes part II. We hope you've enjoyed learning about your chakra type(s) with an eye to making the perfect food choices for you and selecting from among the best ways to enhance your overall health. In part III, based on what you've learned, you'll put together a custom-made plan that will have you glowing in no time.

Part III

BUILDING YOUR CHAKRA MAP

You made it! Now that you're familiar with your chakra type, and you've read the chapters for your strongest chakra and your special, unique twelfth chakra, it's time to put it all together.

It's time to create your customized map to health.

We'll make it simple. All you need is something to write with and access to the questions you answered at the end of your chakra-type chapter.

16

CREATING YOUR PERSONALIZED PLAN

Have you ever written out a health and eating plan? If you have, ours is more fun. You won't need to abide by calories or strict rules. There's no need to log in everything you put in your mouth. Just some flexible guidelines, customized to your chakra type, for you to consider.

In this chapter, you'll pool the information you've learned about eating for your chakra type to create an overall map titled "Chakra Type Map." We'll also provide a range of maps you can employ on a weekly basis that will enable you to fulfill the goals on your overarching chakra map.

Your Chakra Type Map will cover the various areas of interest you explored in part II. To formulate this chakra map—your template for all decision-making—we provide you with another map you can choose to fill out or not: "Chakras I'd Like to Support." This particular map will help you return to your Chakra Type Map to add supplemental information to support other chakras you'd like to strengthen. And, of course, you can rework that Chakra Type Map any time you want.

How are you going to best fulfill the promises you're making to yourself in your Chakra Type Map? Well, you get to the nitty gritty week by week. To assist you in doing this, we've given you several weekly maps to fill out. We encourage you to tackle each of these maps on a weekly basis, so you can put your chakra energy to good use:

- Weekly Meal Plan
- Weekly Supplement List
- Weekly Shopping List
- Weekly Exercise and Movement
- Weekly Supportive Activities

All in all, we've provided you—no, cancel that—you're providing *yourself* with a complete system for better self-care. Place your filled-out sheets wherever you need them: on your refrigerator door, inside a kitchen cabinet, or in your car. Color them. Scan them so you can print out multiple copies. Enjoy each step of achieving a harmonious lifestyle, weight, and life. It's your life to embrace and enjoy!

But first we want to give you a few tips for completing your Chakra Type Map. Ready? *Yes*, you are!

PERMISSION TO BE YOU: HOW MIGHT YOUR TYPE BUILD A PLAN?

You are *you*—totally unique and special. As a member of a chakra type, however, you will approach a project such as sculpting a chakra map in a certain way. Consider our advice.

Manifestor

You've probably already started to implement the ideas covered in your chakra-type description. Let's face it: once you've decided to do something, it's done. Still, take a few notes from these pages to remind yourself of your best-case actions and review them every so often.

Creator

Your wheels have probably already started turning with all the fabulous recipes and food concoctions to create. That is, if you've gotten past the emotions that came up. If you feel emotionally overwhelmed by the daunting task ahead, fill in your maps and then, step by step, implement one change at a time. Think of creative ways to reward yourself for following your plan.

Thinker

These mapping pages were made for you. You'll find places to check boxes, create to-do lists, and organize all your thoughts. Just get out of your head long enough to put pen to paper. If you aren't getting to the task, you might be mentally resisting. No doubt you'll think of a rational excuse for delaying. Push through that and complete the pages. This is where real change can happen.

Relater

You need people. Get started by recruiting a family member or a friend. Then sit down and create your maps together. In this way, you can hold each other accountable. Having another person share in your health plan makes you happy. When possible, use the buddy system while following your plan. Check in with your companion daily or weekly, especially in the beginning. That support will lead to your success—and great health.

Communicator

You may need to talk it through. Once you've done that, you'll likely complete your own research for all facets of your plan. After all, you're the learner type. Since you're tuned in to all things auditory and written, we recommend creating little reminders and lists in your phone. Reading those pop-up reminders will keep you motivated and on track.

Visualizer

First, get a picture in your mind's eye of the outcome you're aiming for. You're a Visualizer, so use that ability! Then watch this future-self move through each aspect of the plan. Note what's working—and if something doesn't look like it will, change up your plan.

You might also want to beautify your mapping sheets. Create a slick design for your plan or place your weekly menu on a well-drawn chalkboard or whiteboard. Using visual cues will draw your future, and your healthiest self, to you.

Spiritualist

Have you meditated on the information in your chapter yet? We're assuming you have. You'll likely need to commune with your identified Higher Power while filling out the chakra-type sheets too. Remember that the goal of these steps is to balance your human and divine selves. So be real about your everyday needs. Then include a couple of cheat foods every so often to make your angelic intentions as practical as possible.

Mystic

We're assuming you may have a hard time deciding which type to go with. *Choose* one and try it for at least three to four weeks. You can always try another type later! Insert our special Mystic chakra–type advice and call a couple of spiritual guides to the task. If you're still struggling to write down a plan, activate your inner Thinker, who loves analytics and project management.

Harmonizer

While filling in your mapping sheets, reflect on the ways you can serve the world. When completing your weekly menu plan, put a star next to the meal you'll make in bulk so you can donate the rest. Look up some local events, farmer's markets, or 5k-runs that support foundations, organizations, causes, and people you care about. If you can't seem to get out of your own idealism, anchor yourself in the Thinker type while creating your map.

Naturalist

Okay, let's be straight up. Avoidance is one of your personality shortcomings. Don't let it get the best of you. Compose your map outdoors. That's right! If it's cold or raining, at least park yourself in front of a window you can gaze through. Remember: you're a member of the natural world. Care for yourself in the same way you care for all natural beings.

Commander

Since you're the boss, you've already had a thousand ideas about how to execute your health plan. Command your own energy and complete the mapping sheets. Then at least entertain the idea of having a staff. Who can do the shopping with your list in hand? Who else can prep with you? Heck, it's okay to be your own leader too.

The Unique You—Your Twelfth Chakra Self

Based on your discoveries in chapter 15 in regard to your twelfth chakra, you now hold some special information about yourself. Why keep it a secret? Go ahead and review your definitive and divine specialties, and think about how they might transfer into a customized health program.

Map Builder Sheets

It's officially time. There are two broad areas of maps for you to fill out so you can continue creating your true-to-your-soul life. As we mentioned earlier, we've organized your map builder sheets into the following two categories: Creating your Chakra Type Map and Weekly Chakra Activities. Please make copies of each map so you can update your Chakra Type Map whenever you desire and fill out the weekly maps on a continual basis.

Ready to seize the day—and your health? Sure you are!

CREATING YOUR CHAKRA TYPE MAP

Fill out the following Chakra Type Map, giving yourself as much time as you need to accomplish this self-loving feat. If you want to account for secondary chakras you'd like to boost, you can complete the worksheet Chakras I'd Like to Support, either before or after completing the Chakra Type Map.

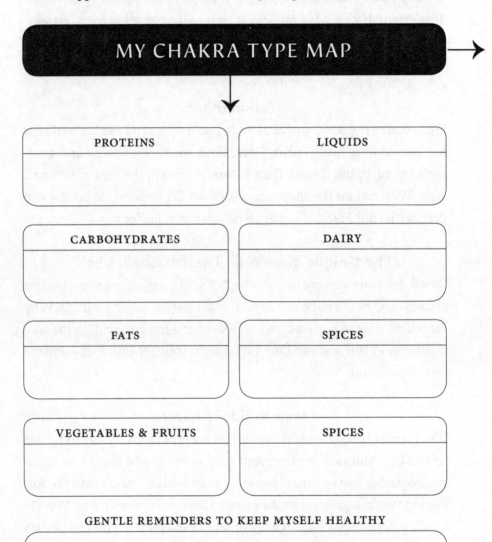

MY CHAKRA TYPE MAP

| PROTEINS | LIQUIDS |

| CARBOHYDRATES | DAIRY |

| FATS | SPICES |

| VEGETABLES & FRUITS | SPICES |

GENTLE REMINDERS TO KEEP MYSELF HEALTHY

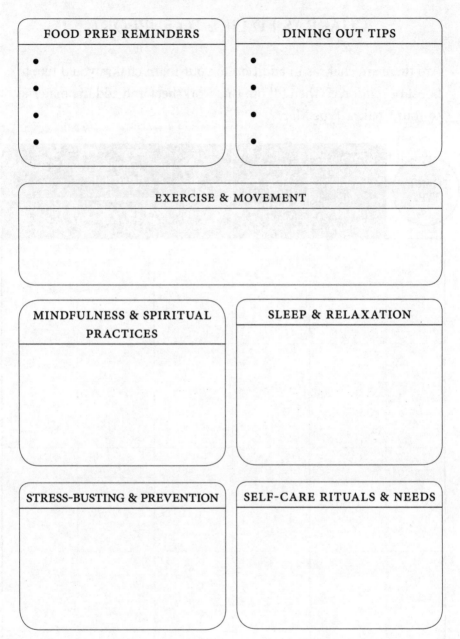

FOOD PREP REMINDERS

-
-
-
-

DINING OUT TIPS

-
-
-
-

EXERCISE & MOVEMENT

MINDFULNESS & SPIRITUAL PRACTICES

SLEEP & RELAXATION

STRESS-BUSTING & PREVENTION

SELF-CARE RITUALS & NEEDS

CHAKRAS I'D LIKE TO SUPPORT

Are there are chakras in addition to your main chakra you'd like to boost or reinforce? Then fill out this worksheet and add the material to your Chakra Type Map.

CHAKRA TYPE	WHY DO I WANT TO SUPPORT THIS CHAKRA TYPE?	WHAT AM I LOOKING TO DEVELOP WITHIN MYSELF?	HOW I'D LIKE TO SUPPORT THIS CHAKRA THROUGH:		
			FOOD, LIQUIDS, & SPICES	SUPPLEMENTS	SUPPORTIVE ACTIVITY

WEEKLY CHAKRA ACTIVITIES

We're providing you with several worksheets to fill out on a weekly basis. These are based on your already-completed Chakra Type Map. They will enable you to fulfill your goals of harmony and joy.

Weekly Meal Plan

What's up for dining this week? Make your decisions here.

	BREAKFAST	LUNCH	DINNER	SNACKS
MONDAY				
TUESDAY				
WEDNESDAY				
THURSDAY				
FRIDAY				
SATURDAY				
SUNDAY				

Weekly Supplements List

What supplements support your body's needs? Plan out your supplements protocol here.

	SUPPLEMENTS
MONDAY	
TUESDAY	
WEDNESDAY	
THURSDAY	
FRIDAY	
SATURDAY	
SUNDAY	

SUPPLEMENTS TO PURCHASE

☐   ☐

☐   ☐

☐   ☐

☐   ☐

Weekly Shopping List

Ready to shop! Do it your way (and resist the *Nopes!*)

	ITEMS TO BUY		
PROTEINS	☐ ☐ ☐	☐ ☐ ☐	☐ ☐ ☐
CARBOHYDRATES	☐ ☐ ☐	☐ ☐ ☐	☐ ☐ ☐
FATS	☐ ☐ ☐	☐ ☐ ☐	☐ ☐ ☐
VEGETABLES & FRUITS	☐ ☐ ☐	☐ ☐ ☐	☐ ☐ ☐
LIQUIDS	☐ ☐ ☐	☐ ☐ ☐	☐ ☐ ☐
DAIRY	☐ ☐ ☐	☐ ☐ ☐	☐ ☐ ☐
SPICES	☐ ☐ ☐	☐ ☐ ☐	☐ ☐ ☐
SNACKS	☐ ☐ ☐	☐ ☐ ☐	☐ ☐ ☐
SUPPLEMENTS	☐ ☐ ☐	☐ ☐ ☐	☐ ☐ ☐

Weekly Exercise & Movement

What movements call to you this week? Chart out how and when you want to move your body.

	EXERCISE	TIME OF DAY	LOCATION	GOAL
MONDAY				
TUESDAY				
WEDNESDAY				
THURSDAY				
FRIDAY				
SATURDAY				
SUNDAY				

Weekly Supportive Activities

Life is meant to be fully lived. What better way to live your life to the fullest than to support yourself every inch of the way?

	FOOD PREP REMINDERS	DINING OUT TIPS	MINDFULNESS & SPIRITUAL PRACTICES	SLEEP & RELAXATION	STRESS-BUSTING & PREVENTION	SELF-CARE RITUALS & NEEDS
MONDAY						
TUESDAY						
WEDNESDAY						
THURSDAY						
FRIDAY						
SATURDAY						
SUNDAY						

YOU'RE ALL SET!

How does it feel? You have a brand-new plan tailored to who you are right now. Remember that, at any time, you can revisit the quiz and the types. After all, you're human and you'll evolve.

Taking the quiz periodically allows you to be conscious of your evolution. How about keeping an updated plan? Maybe that's what New Year's Eve could be for, or the eve before your birthday?

Completing the quiz and maps at a set time on a periodic basis ensures that you are constantly supporting yourself. It's also a great way to watch your progression. What if you have an important event coming up? How about a new job, or anything else that requires you show up differently? It's time to look over the types again. In that list, you're bound to find a type that embodies the qualities you're seeking. Put suggestions from that chosen type into your map, even if only for a short while. You'll be prepared for your event and the better for it.

Remember: above all, you're the one who knows you best. (Even better now that you have taken the quiz and know your type.) Honor who you are and only plug ideas into your map that really suit you. This is your life, and it really does get to be all about you.

ACKNOWLEDGMENTS

We had so much help with this book, both personally and professionally.

We want to thank the editors and staff at St. Martin's Press, including Elizabeth Beier and Hannah Phillips, and the agents who helped bring this to life: Coleen O'Shea and Anthony J. W. Benson. Thank you to Glenn Chappell, for working diligently with us on the creation of the beautiful chakra-type icons. And a massive thanks to Sheridan McCarthy of Meadowlark Publishing Services, our editing champion.

Dana: A book cannot be written in isolation. There is so much love, support, and help that pours in. Here, I thank a portion of all those who supported me.

Cyndi, you have been the greatest writing partner. Sharing in the pain and joy and pushing it forward with your notorious lightning speed. May the powers of progesterone always be at our beck and call. Sufi, for your endless reminders to take a break, go for a walk, and make time to play with friends. Noah, thanks for being you and an endless source of heart opening; the world is lucky to have you.

Thank you to my mold cleaning support team: Jacob, Holly, Amy, Jenny B, Meghan, Meg W., Grace, Ann H., CJ, Rebecca, Nicole, Nikki E., Rochelle, Brooke, Susan, Emily, Caroline, Debbie, Hilary, Johanna, Sarah, Maria, and Jane. And thanks to my mold emotional support team: Terri Matthews, Nicole Broadus, Laurie Anderson, and

Meg Reynolds. And to my mold chef for all the food love, Patti Bryan. Woman, you are a food Goddess and my hero.

Thank you to Goop, especially Kelly, Kiki, and Élise for the agent connection and the support. And to my moral support team, Jacob Stohler and Jim Yost. You guys were right, hope floats. Special love to The Sisterhood of the Traveling Pens, who helped me believe writing a book was possible. Special thanks to Amelia, Debbie, and Wendy for allowing us to work on this during our Pilgrimage. Unending gratitude for Sufi's second family, The Milgates, and for Anne who gave me hope and a place to live. Thank you to Amy Langdon and Audrey Mercer, who keep my social media moving, and to Emily Serenius, whom I am eternally grateful for. Katie Craig, my web wizard, my gratitude is unending for your tech prowess; thank you for keeping me (mostly) sane. And to Sarah Gargano and India Gentile, for all the PR savvy. To Lee Staley, my video and sound editing man, you are a Godsend.

Last, but certainly not least, thank you to my family. Mom and Dad, I am ever so fortunate to call you my parents and to have learned how to listen to and chase my own heart because of your influence. To Misti, for accepting that I'm the favorite and for being the funny one. I love you. To Denise, thank you for being a light in the dark for those you serve.

Cyndi: How could I not give my hugest hug of thanks to Dana? Our partnership is about more than writing, it's about friendship and true care. Balancing Dana's little Yoda-like Sufi-dog are my two hulks, Honey the Golden Retriever and Lucky the yellow Lab, who never let me forget that the true meaning of life is food.

To the next stage of professional fun, I thank my publicity team, Steve Allen Media. Hats off to Steve, Mara, Amanda, Ashley, and Angela. We keep each other busy! And MPulse Communications, my extraordinaire social media team. I'm actually starting to get the hang of all this posting!

THANKS A TON to my friends Julie and JJ, women of wisdom, my great friend Donny, and my special Saturday night group consisting of Pam, Wendy, Jeff, Kris, and many spiritual assistants. Another ode (as one was already lovingly made by Dana) to the El Camino gals: Dana, Wendy, Debbie, and Amelia. And my rock-solid healers, Ofer, Michele, and Cindy, who keep me honest and not complaining too much. Finally, who would I be without my kids? Michael and his partner Lianne, whose adventures keep carrying them higher in the world, and my son Gabe, who throws a baseball higher and faster than I could toss a super ball. All love to them, my clients and students, and a blessing for Hope for All.

BIBLIOGRAPHY

INTRODUCTION

Lipton, Bruce. *The Biology of Belief*. Carlsbad, CA: Hay House, 2008.

Woodroffe, Sir John (Arthur Avalon). *The Serpent Power*. Mineola, NY: Dover, 1974 (first published in 1919). https://www.bhagavadgitausa.com/Serpent%20Power%20Complete.pdf

3. PRACTICAL TIPS ON FOODSTUFFS FOR ALL CHAKRA TYPES

Axe, Josh. "The 5 Worst Artificial Sweeteners, Plus Healthy Alternatives." *Dr. Axe*, March 21, 2018. https://draxe.com/nutrition/artificial-sweeteners/

4. MANIFESTOR

Campbell, Becky. "Exactly What to Eat (and What to Avoid) to Eliminate Stress and Support Your Adrenals." *Mindbodygreen*, July 19, 2017. http://www.mindbodygreen.com/articles/the-best-foods-for-adrenal-support

Eller, Ericka. "What Do I Eat If I Have Adrenal Fatigue?" November 20, 2018. http://www.erickaeller.com/blog/2018/10/19/what-do-i-eat-if-i-have-adrenal-fatigue

Fischer, Christie. "Weird and Wacky Nutrition for Adrenal Fatigue." September 17, 2013. http://www.christiefischer.com/2013/09/weird-and-whacky-nutrition-for-adrenal.html

Goldman, Leslie. "Is It Adrenal Fatigue?" *Yoga Journal*, November 14, 2018. http://www.yogajournal.com/poses/adrenal-fatigue-tired

Hansen, Fawne. "Should You Avoid Alcohol If You Have Adrenal Fatigue?" *The Adrenal Solution*, January 1, 2017. https://adrenalfatiguesolution.com/alcohol-adrenal-fatigue/

Mawer, Randy. "Hemp Protein Powder: The Best Plant-Based Protein?" *Healthline*, August 4, 2018. https://www.healthline.com/nutrition/hemp-protein-powder#bottom-line

Cording, Jess. "Urban Remedy's Neka Pasquale on Making Health Delicious," *Forbes*, March 5, 2018. https://www.forbes.com/sites/jesscording/2018/03/05/urban-remedy-neka -pasquale/?sh=6f13e6e74163

Strawbridge, Holly. "Artificial Sweeteners: Sugar-Free, but at What Cost?" Harvard Medical School, January 29, 2020. http://www.health.harvard.edu/blog/artificial-sweeteners -sugar-free-but-at-what-cost-201207165030

"The Sweet Danger of Sugar." *Harvard Health Men's Watch*, November 5, 2019. https:// www.health.harvard.edu/heart-health/the-sweet-danger-of-sugar

"What Is Cortisol?" *WebMD*, December 22, 2018. http://www.webmd.com/a-to-z-guides /what-is-cortisol#1

Wilson, James L. "Foods to Eat and Foods to Avoid for Adrenal Fatigue." *AdrenalFatigue .org*, July 18, 2018. https://adrenalfatigue.org/foods-eat-avoid-adrenal-fatigue/

5. Creator

ADVANCE staff. "Improving Endocrine Health Through a Healthy Diet." *Elite Health-care*, March 12, 2018. https://www.elitecme.com/resource-center/nursing/improving -endocrine-health-through-a-healthy-diet

"The Best Vitamins and Supplements for Male Reproductive System." *WonderLabs*, December 7, 2017. https://www.wonderlabs.com/blog/the-best-vitamins-and-supplements -for-male-reproductive-system

Bouchez, Colette. "The Six Super Foods Every Woman Needs." *WebMD*, November 19, 2008. https://www.webmd.com/women/features/six-super-foods-every-woman-needs#1

Elist, James. "Five Vitamins for Male Sexual Health." *Dr. Elist MD Facts*. https://www .drelist.com/blog/vitamins-male-sexual-health/

Furness, John B. "Enteric Nervous System." *Scholarpedia* 2(10), August 23, 2007:4064. http://www.scholarpedia.org/article/Enteric_nervous_system

Johnson, Jackie. "Tips on Balancing the Sacral Chaka." *Herbal Academy*, June 27, 2016. https://theherbalacademy.com/tips-on-balancing-the-sacral-chakra/

Kubala, Jillian. "Is Saturated Fat Unhealthy?" *Healthline*, March 25, 2020. https://www .healthline.com/nutrition/saturated-fat#what-it-is

Mawer, Randy. "The 8 Best Supplements to Boost Testosterone Levels." *Healthline*, September 2, 2016. https://www.healthline.com/nutrition/best-testosterone-booster -supplements#section1

Olson, Natalie. "20 Foods Rich in Selenium." *Healthline*, April 15, 2019. https://www .healthline.com/health/selenium-foods#brown-rice

Santilli, Mara. "The Best Types of Food to Eat and Avoid When You Have PCOS." *CCRM Fertility*, May 13, 2019. https://www.ccrmivf.com/news-events/food-pcos/

Tremblay, Sylvie. "Food for Healthy Ovaries." *SFGate,* December 2, 2018. https://healthyeating.sfgate.com/food-healthy-ovaries-9841.html

"What to Eat for Testicular Health." *New Hope Unlimited.* https://www.newhopemedical center.com/blogs/what-to-eat-for-testicular-health/

6. THINKER

"Best and Worst Foods for Pancreatitis Pain." Cleveland Clinic, March 23, 2020. https://health.clevelandclinic.org/best-and-worst-foods-for-pancreatitis-pain/

"Carbohydrates and Blood Sugar." Harvard T. H. Chan School of Public Health, 2020. https://www.hsph.harvard.edu/nutritionsource/carbohydrates/carbohydrates-and-blood-sugar/

Chandler, Stephanie. "High-Protein Diet and the Pancreas." *Livestrong.* https://www.livestrong.com/article/547754-high-protein-diet-and-the-pancreas/

"5 Foods That Improve Pancreatic Health." *Randox Health*, December 28, 2016. https://medium.com/@RandoxHealth/5-foods-that-improve-pancreatic-health-9509e241911

George, Katherine. "Foods That Promote a Healthy Pancreas." *Active Beat*, May 19, 2020. https://www.activebeat.com/diet-nutrition/8-eats-for-a-healthy-pancreas/

Gerszberg, Deborah. "Help Take Pain Out of Pancreatitis with Your Diet." *Clinical Nutritionist,* The Pancreas Center, Columbia Surgery.org. https://columbiasurgery.org/news/2013/04/11/help-take-pain-out-pancreatitis-your-diet

McDougall, John. "The Pancreas—Under Attack by Cow-Milk." *Vegan Lifestyle Coach*, July 2002. https://www.veganlifestylecoach.com/dairy-and-the-pancreas

"Nutrition Advice and Recipes." The National Pancreas Foundation. https://pancreas foundation.org/patient-information/nutrition-advice-recipes/

"The 12 Best Foods & Herbs for a Healthy Pancreas." *Mediterranean Hospital.* https://www.medihospital.com.cy/robotics/blog/78-the-12-best-foods-herbs-for-a-healthy-pancreas

7. RELATER

"Blood Vessels." The Franklin Institute. https://www.fi.edu/heart/blood-vessels

Boham, Elizabeth. "My Top 5 Supplements for Breast Health." *The Ultrawellness Center*, October 18, 2018. https://www.ultrawellnesscenter.com/2018/10/18/my-top-5-supplements-for-breast-health/

Brunet. "9 Food Combinations That Offer Incredible Benefits." Brunet. https://www.brunet.ca/en/health/health-tips/9-food-combinations-that-offer-incredible-health-benefits/

Dairy Nutrition. "Cardiovascular Disease and Milk Products: Summary of Evidence." Dairy Nutrition. https://www.dairynutrition.ca/scientific-evidence/cardiovascular-disease/cardiovascular-disease-and-milk-products-summary-of-evidence

"8 Heart Supplements to Take—and One to Avoid." *Healthy You,* January 30, 2018. https://www.peacehealth.org/healthy-you/8-heart-health-supplements-take-and-one-avoid

Errey, Sally. "Food Combinations for a Healthy Heart." Alive, April 24, 2015. https://www.alive.com/food/food-combinations-for-a-healthy-heart/

Nathan Yueh et al., "New Insights Into Heart Healthy Dietary Habits: What the Clinician Needs to Know," American College of Cardiology, March 27, 2020. https://www.acc.org/latest-in-cardiology/articles/2020/03/27/09/04/new-insights-into-heart-healthy-dietary-habits#:~:text=Per%20the%20ACC%2FAHA%20and,per%20week)%20have%20additional%20benefits

"Heart of the Matter: 4 Heart Health Supplements Backed by Science." *Care/of.* https://takecareof.com/articles/guide-to-heart-health

Link, Rachel. "15 Incredibly Heart-Healthy Foods." *Healthline,* March 5, 2018. https://www.healthline.com/nutrition/heart-healthy-foods

Mayo Clinic Staff. "Heart-Healthy Diet." Mayo Clinic. https://www.mayoclinic.org/diseases-conditions/heart-disease/in-depth/heart-healthy-diet/art-20047702

Mayo Clinic Staff. "Mediterranean Diet: A Heart-Healthy Eating Plan." Mayo Clinic. https://www.mayoclinic.org/healthy-lifestyle/nutrition-and-healthy-eating/in-depth/mediterranean-diet/art-20047801

McCraty, Rollin. "The Heart-Brain Connection." HeartMath. https://www.heartmath.com/science/

Sager, Jeanne. "Heart-Healthy Food Combinations." Sheknows, January 2, 2010. https://www.sheknows.com/food-and-recipes/articles/812910/heart-healthy-food-combinations/

Sheikh, Anees, ed. *Healing Images: The Role of Imagination in Health.* Amityville, New York: Baywood Publishing Company, 2003.

"Stocking a Heart-Healthy Kitchen." Cleveland Clinic, updated July 17, 2019. https://my.clevelandclinic.org/health/articles/11916-stocking-a-heart-healthy-kitchen

Storrs, Carina. "Vitamin E May Protect the Lungs." Explore Health, May 16, 2010. https://www.health.com/condition/smoking/vitamin-e-lungs

Suglia, Shakira, Katherine J.Sapra, and Karestan C. Koenen. "Violence and Cardiovascular Health: A Systematic Review." *American Journal of Preventive Medicine*, 48(2): February 2015, 205–12. https://www.ncbi.nlm.nih.gov/pmc/articles/PMC4300436/

Thomassian, Melanie. "Drink to Your Health." *Healthcentral,* July 28, 2008. https://www.healthcentral.com/article/drink-to-your-heart-top-10-beverages-to-keep-your-heart-healthy

8. COMMUNICATOR

CHI St. Luke's Health. "5 Foods That Improve Thyroid Function." January 12, 2018. https://www.chistlukeshealth.org/resources/5-foods-improve-thyroid-function

"Foods That Help or Hurt Your Thyroid." *WebMD,* November 5, 2019. https://www.webmd
.com/women/manage-hypothyroidism-17/balance/slideshow-foods-thyroid

Healthbeat. "Healthy Eating for a Healthy Thyroid." Harvard Medical School. https://www
.health.harvard.edu/staying-healthy/healthy-eating-for-a-healty-thyroid

Liao, Sharon. "Exercises for an Underactive Thyroid." *WebMD,* December 1, 2017. https://
www.webmd.com/women/manage-hypothyroidism-17/balance/exercises-underactive
-thyroid

Natural Endocrine Solutions. "The Truth About Protein, Carbs, Fats, & Thyroid Health."
https://www.naturalendocrinesolutions.com/articles/truth-protein-carbs-fats-thyroid
-health/

Raman, Ryan. "Best Diet for Hypothyroidism: Foods to Eat, Foods to Avoid." *Healthline,*
November 15, 2019. https://www.healthline.com/nutrition/hypothyroidism-diet

Shomon, Mary. "Nutrition Tips for Thyroid Patients." *Verywell Health,* August 5, 2020.
https://www.verywellhealth.com/nutrition-tips-for-thyroid-wellness-4067153

Thompson, Dennis, Jr. "9 Foods to Avoid If You're Diagnosed with Hypothyrodism."
Everyday Health, January 30, 2020. https://www.everydayhealth.com/hs/thyroid
-pictures/foods-to-avoid/

Valpone, Amie. "Why You Need Carbs for a Healthy Thyroid, Metabolism, & Adrenals."
The Healthy Apple, October 19, 2015. https://thehealthyapple.com/why-you-need-carbs
-for-a-healthy-thyroid-metabolism-adrenals/

9. Visualizer
Abbot, Jo. "Chemical Messengers: How Our Hormones Help Us Sleep." *The Conversation,*
September 9, 2015. https://theconversation.com/chemical-messengers-how-hormones
-help-us-sleep-44983

Brown, Mary Jane. "Monk Fruit Sweetener: Good or Bad?" *Healthline,* June 14, 2019.
https://www.healthline.com/nutrition/monk-fruit-sweetener#benefits

Cadman, Bethany. "How to Remove Cortisol from the Body Naturally." *Medical News
Today,* January 15, 2020. https://www.medicalnewstoday.com/articles/322335#natural
-ways-to-lower-cortisol

Gunnars, Kris. "Intermittent Fasting 101—The Ultimate Beginner's Guide." *Healthline,*
April 20, 2020. https://www.healthline.com/nutrition/intermittent-fasting-guide#effects

"Exercising to Relax." *Harvard Men's Health Watch,* February 2011. https://www.health
.harvard.edu/staying-healthy/exercising-to-relax

McGrane, Kelli. "13 Nearly Complete Protein Sources for Vegetarians and Vegans."
Healthline. April 21, 2020. https://www.healthline.com/nutrition/complete-protein
-for-vegans

Meng Xiao, Ya Li, Sha Li, Yue Zhou, Ren-You Gan, Dong-Ping Xu, and Hua-Bin Li. "Dietary

Sources and Bioactivities of Melatonin." *Nutrients*, April 2017, 9(4):367. https://www.ncbi.nlm.nih.gov/pmc/articles/PMC5409706/

Rachdaoui, Nadia, and Dipak Sarkar. "Effects of Alcohol on the Endocrine System." *Endocrinology and Metabolism Clinics of North America*, September 2013, 42(3):593–615. https://www.ncbi.nlm.nih.gov/pmc/articles/PMC3767933/

Raman, Ryan. "Top 11 Benefits of Bee Pollen." *Healthline*, August 13, 2018. https://www.healthline.com/nutrition/bee-pollen

West, Helen. "How Artificial Sweeteners Affect Blood Sugar and Insulin." *Healthline*, June 3, 2017. https://www.healthline.com/nutrition/artificial-sweeteners-blood-sugar-insulin

"Your Hormones." The Pituitary Foundation. 2018. https://www.pituitary.org.uk/information/hormones/

10. SPIRITUALIST

Coyle, Daisy, APD. "7 Foods That Still Contain Trans Fats." *Healthline*, October 29, 2018. https://www.healthline.com/nutrition/trans-fat-foods

Duggal, Neel. "5 Functions of the Pineal Gland." *Healthline*, April 7, 2017. https://www.healthline.com/health/pineal-gland-function#tips

Huizen, Jennifer. "Which Foods Can Help You Sleep?" *Medical News Today*, January 25, 2019. https://www.medicalnewstoday.com/articles/324295

Knott, Laurence. "Pineal Gland and Circadian Rhythms." *Patient,* December 19, 2016. https://patient.info/doctor/pineal-gland-and-circadian-rhythms#:~:text=In%20the%20absence%20of%20light,Endocrine%20rhythms

Korkmaz, Ahmet, Russel J. Reiter, Dun-Xian Tan, and Lucien C. Manchester. "Melotonin: From Pineal Gland to Healthy Foods." Spatula DD 1, 2011:33–36. https://pdfs.semanticscholar.org/3ec4/476ef327d4480b1c9d152ce6636ac467a551.pdf

Peuhkuri, Katri, Nora Sihvola, and Riitta Korpela. "Dietary Factors and Fluctuating Levels of Melatonin." *Food & Nutrition Research* 56, July 20, 2012. https://www.ncbi.nlm.nih.gov/pmc/articles/PMC3402070/

Raypole, Crystal. "6 Ways to Boost Serotonin Without Medication." *Healthline*, April 22, 2019. https://www.healthline.com/health/how-to-increase-serotonin#diet

Sissons, Claire. "How to Boost Serotonin and Improve Mood." *Medical News Today*, July 10, 2018. https://www.medicalnewstoday.com/articles/322416

"3 Strategies to Fight Seasonal Affective Disorder." Cleveland Health Clinic, November 12, 2019. https://health.clevelandclinic.org/3-best-strategies-help-fight-seasonal-affective-disorder/

11. MYSTIC

Bailey, Joshua. "How to Increase the Thymus Function." *Livestrong.* https://www.livestrong.com/article/548758-how-to-increase-the-thymus-function/

Beychok, Tina. "Simple Ways to Strengthen Your Thymus Gland." *Chiropractic Economics*, May 11, 2018. https://www.chiroeco.com/thymus-supplement/

Dworkin, Michael. "Boosting the Immune System with Natural Remedies" (Part I). *Natural Nutmeg*, November 10, 2016. https://naturalnutmeg.com/boosting-the-immune-system-with-natural-remedies-part-1/

Goldstein, Valerie. "Immune System: The Gut, Thymus and Bone Marrow (Part 3 of 3) Fight for Health." *Eating Fuel to Health*. https://eatingtofuelhealth.com/fight-for-health/

Hill, Steve. "Dr. Greg Fahy—Rejuvenating the Thymus to Prevent Age-Related Disease." *Life Extension Advocacy*, October 4, 2017. https://www.lifespan.io/news/rejuvenating-the-thymus/

Maffetone, Phil. "The Many Benefits of Dietary Fat." *MAF,* December 10, 2016. https://philmaffetone.com/benefits-of-dietary-fat/

Mein, Carolyn. "The Thymus Body Type." The 25 Body Type System. https://bodytype.com/bodytypes/thymus_body_type.php

Parla, Jayagopal. "Ayurveda's Answer to How to Improve Your Immune System." *Sonima,* December 18, 2017. https://www.sonima.com/food/health-nutrition/maintaining-good-health/

Sheldrick, Giles. "Secret Anti-Aging Remedy Revealed—and It's in Your FRIDGE." *Express,* August 7, 2015. https://www.express.co.uk/life-style/diets/596642/anti-aging-remedy-fridge-diet-food-research

12. Harmonizer

Bjarnadottir, Adda. "13 Foods That Cause Bloating and What to Eat Instead." *Healthline*, June 4, 2017. https://www.healthline.com/nutrition/13-foods-that-cause-bloating

Greenspan, Noah. *Ultimate Pulmonary Wellness.* New York: Pulmonary Wellness and Rehabilitation Center, 2017.

Hadjiliadis, Denis, Paul F. Harron, Jr., David Zieve, and A.D.A.M. Editorial team. "Diaphragm and Lungs." *Medline Plus Medical Encyclopedia*, May 16, 2019. https://medlineplus.gov/ency/imagepages/19380.htm

Huizen, Jennifer. "Vitamins and Supplements for Increased Blood Flow." *Medical News Today*, July 23, 2019. https://www.medicalnewstoday.com/articles/325829

Kitaoka, Hiroko, and Koji Chihara. "The Diaphragm: A Hidden but Essential Organ for the Mammal and the Human." *Advances in Experimental Medicine and Biology*, December 2010, 669:167–71. https://pubmed.ncbi.nlm.nih.gov/20217342/

Moyer, Nancy, L. "Why Do I Hiccup After Eating?" *Healthline*, November 26, 2018. https://www.healthline.com/health/hiccups-after-eating

Mpatino, "Foods to Avoid with COPD." Lung Health Institute, May 1, 2014. https://lunginstitute.com/blog/foods-to-avoid-with-copd/

Norton, Amy. "Diet Tied to Better Breathing in COPD Patients." *WebMD*, May 21, 2014. https://www.webmd.com/lung/news/20140521/diet-tied-to-better-breathing-in-copd -patients

Romieu, Isabelle. "Nutrition and Lung Health." *The International Journal of Tuberculosis and Lung Disease*, April 2005, 9(4):362–74. https://www.ncbi.nlm.nih.gov/pubmed /15830741

"10 Tips for Eating When You Have Breathing Problems." *WebMD*, October 24, 2018. https://www.webmd.com/lung/tips-eating-breathing-problems

"Understanding Heartburn—Prevention." *WebMD*, January 24, 2020. https://www.webmd .com/heartburn-gerd/guide/understanding-heartburn-prevention

Wax, Emily, David Zieve, and A.D.A.M. Editorial team. "Facts About Polyunsaturated Fats." Medline Plus Medical Encyclopedia, April 23, 2018. https://medlineplus.gov /ency/patientinstructions/000747.htm

13. NATURALIST

Bonjour, Jean-Philippe. "Dietary Protein: An Essential Nutrient for Bone Health." *PubMed*, December 2005. https://pubmed.ncbi.nlm.nih.gov/16373952/

"By the Way, Doctor, Does Carbonated Water Harm Bones?" *Harvard Women's Health Watch*, January 2010, updated April 16, 2019. https://www.health.harvard.edu/staying -healthy/does-carbonated-water-harm-bones

Domazetovic, Vladana, Gemma Marcucci, Teresa Iantomasi, Maria Luisa Brandi, and Maria Teresa Vincenzini. "Oxidative Stress in Bone Remodeling: Role of Antioxidants." *Clinical Cases in Mineral and Bone Metabolism*, May–August 2017, 14(2):209–16. https://www.ncbi.nlm.nih.gov/pmc/articles/PMC5726212/

Heaney, Robert P., and Donald K. Layman. "Amount and type of protein influences bone health." *The American Journal of Clinical Nutrition*, May 1, 2008;87(5). https:// academic.oup.com/ajcn/article/87/5/1567S/4650438

Layne, J. E., and M. E. Nelson. "The effects of progressive resistance training on bone density: a review." *Medical and Science in Sports and Exercise*, December 31, 1998, 31(1): 25–30. https://europepmc.org/article/med/9927006

Moser, Sarah C., and Bram C. J. van der Eerden. "Osteocalcin—A Versatile Bone-Derived Hormone." *Frontiers in Endocrinology*. January 10, 2019. https://www.frontiersin.org /articles/10.3389/fendo.2018.00794/full

Neustadt, John. "Top Alkaline Foods to Eat & Acid Foods to Avoid." *NBI Health*. https:// nbihealth.com/top-alkaline-foods-to-eat-acid-foods-to-avoid/

"Vitamin C." *Medline Plus Medical Encyclopedia*, June 2, 2020. https://medlineplus.gov /ency/article/002404.htm

14. COMMANDER

Asboe-Hansen, G. "Season Effects on Connective Tissue." *American Physiological Reviews*, July 1, 1958. https://journals.physiology.org/doi/abs/10.1152/physrev.1958.38.3.446 ?journalCode=physrev

"Characteristics of Connective Tissue." *Lumen*. https://courses.lumenlearning.com /boundless-ap/chapter/connective-tissue/

Steve Grant Health. "Nutrition strategies for connective tissue injury prevention and recovery." https://www.stevegranthealth.com/articles/nutrition-strategies-connective -tissue-injury-prevention-recovery/

Eller, Esther, review. "4 Keys to Strength Building and Muscle Mass." Academy of Nutrition and Dietetics, January 20, 2020. https://www.eatright.org/fitness/training-and -recovery/building-muscle/strength-building-and-muscle-mass

"Herbs for Healing and Strengthening Connective Tissue." *Herban Wellness*, August 8, 2018. https://www.herbanwellness.net/2018/08/08/herbs-for-healing-and-strengthening -connective-tissue/

The Histology Guide. "Exocrine and Endocrine Glands." University of Leeds. https://www .histology.leeds.ac.uk/glandular/exocr_endocr_properties.php

Hougaard, Rasmus, and Jacqueline Carter. "Senior Executives Get More Sleep Than Everyone Else." *Harvard Business Review*, February 28, 2018. https://hbr.org/2018/02/senior -executives-get-more-sleep-than-everyone-else

Leal, Darla. "Nutrition for Your Muscle Growth." *Verywellfit*, January 13, 2020. https:// www.verywellfit.com/are-you-eating-for-muscle-3121316

Muscle and Fitness Editors. "Top 7 Sources of Carbs to Build Muscle." *Muscle and Fitness*. https://www.muscleandfitness.com/flexonline/flex-nutrition/7-best-carbs-build-muscle/

"The Muscle Matrix Workout to Strengthen Your Connective Tissue." *Muscle and Fitness*. https://www.muscleandfitness.com/routine/workouts/workout-routines/muscle -matrix-workout/

NFPT Team. "Connective Tissue Training." National Federation of Professional Trainers, February 13, 2015. https://www.nfpt.com/blog/connective-tissue-training

"Nutrition Strategies for Connective Tissue Injury Prevention and Recovery." *Steve Grant Health*. https://www.stevegranthealth.com/articles/nutrition-strategies-connective -tissue-injury-prevention-recovery/

Owen, Buffy. "Nourishing Your Connective Tissue with Whole Foods." *Conscious Movements*. https://www.consciousmovements.com/body-mind-blog/nourish-your-tissue -with-whole-foods

Padarin, Helen. "Nutrition for Healthy Connective Tissue." May 11, 2017. https://helenpadarin .com/uncategorised/nutrition-healthy-connective-tissue/

Tinsley, Grant. "The 6 Best Supplements to Gain Muscle." *Healthline*, July 16, 2017. https://
www.healthline.com/nutrition/supplements-for-muscle-gain

Tinsley, Grant. "26 Foods That Help You Build Lean Muscle." *Healthline*, January 21, 2018.
https://www.healthline.com/nutrition/26-muscle-building-foods

Tozzi, Paolo. "Does Fascia Hold Memories?" Fascia Science and Clinical Applications.
Journal of Bodywork & Movement Therapies, April 1, 2014, 18(2):259–65. https://
pubmed.ncbi.nlm.nih.gov/24725795/

Tupler, Julie. "Find Out Why Nutrition Is Important for Healing Your Connective Tissue."
Tupler Technique, April 22, 2020. https://diastasisrehab.com/blogs/news/importance
-of-nutrition-for-healing-connective-tissue

ABOUT THE AUTHOR

Cyndi Dale is an internationally renowned author, speaker, intuitive healer, and visionary. She is president of Life Systems Services, a corporation that offers intuitive-based healing, destiny coaching, and corporate consulting. She is the author of twenty-seven highly acclaimed books about energy medicine, intuition, and holistic healing. She lives in Minneapolis with her family.

Dana Childs is an intuitive, energy healer, teacher, and speaker. She leads workshops, online courses, and retreats to help you access your true self and open your intuitive gifts. She lives with her dog, Sufi, in North Carolina.